PET-Based Interventions

Editor

RAKESH KUMAR

PET CLINICS

www.pet.theclinics.com

Consulting Editor
ABASS ALAVI

October 2015 • Volume 10 • Number 4

ELSEVIER

1600 John F. Kennedy Boulevard • Suite 1800 • Philadelphia, Pennsylvania, 19103-2899

http://www.pet.theclinics.com

PET CLINICS Volume 10, Number 4
October 2015 ISSN 1556-8598, ISBN-13: 978-0-323-40100-5

Editor: John Vassallo (j.vassallo@elsevier.com)
Developmental Editor: Meredith Clinton

PET Clinics (ISSN 1556-8598) is published quarterly by Elsevier Inc., 360 Park Avenue South, New York, NY 10010-1710. Months of issue are January, April, July, and October. Periodicals postage paid at New York, NY, and additional mailing offices. Subscription prices per year are $225.00 (US individuals), $327.00 (US institutions), $115.00 (US students), $255.00 (Canadian individuals), $369.00 (Canadian institutions), $140.00 (Canadian students), $275.00 (foreign individuals), $369.00 (foreign institutions), and $140.00 (foreign students). To receive student and resident rate, orders must be accompanied by name of affiliated institution, date of term, and the signature of program/residency coordinator on institution letterhead. Orders will be billed at individual rate until proof of status is received. Foreign air speed delivery is included in all Clinics subscription prices. All prices are subject to change without notice. POSTMASTER: Send address changes to PET Clinics, Elsevier Health Sciences Division, Subscription Customer Service, 3251 Riverport Lane, Maryland Heights, MO 63043. **Customer Service: 1-800-654-2452 (U.S. and Canada); 314-447-8871 (outside U.S. and Canada). Fax: 314-447-8029. E-mail:** journalscustomerservice-usa@elsevier.com **(for print support);** journalsonlinesupport-usa@elsevier.com **(for online support).**

Reprints. For copies of 100 or more of articles in this publication, please contact the Commercial Reprints Department, Elsevier Inc., 360 Park Avenue South, New York, NY 10010-1710. Tel.: 212-633-3874; Fax: 212-633-3820; E-mail: reprints@elsevier.com.

PET Clinics is covered in MEDLINE/PubMed (Index Medicus).

Contributors

CONSULTING EDITOR

ABASS ALAVI, MD, PhD (Hon), Dsc (Hon)
Professor of Radiology, Division of Nuclear
Medicine, Department of Radiology, University
of Pennsylvania School of Medicine, Hospital
of the University of Pennsylvania, Philadelphia,
Pennsylvania

EDITOR

RAKESH KUMAR, MD, PhD
Professor and Head, Diagnostic Nuclear
Medicine Division, Department of Nuclear
Medicine, All India Institute of Medical
Sciences, New Delhi, India

AUTHORS

AHMAD ESMAEEL ABDULLAH, MD
Department of Nuclear Medicine, La Timone
University Hospital, Aix-Marseille University,
Marseille, France

ABASS ALAVI, MD, PhD (Hon), Dsc (Hon)
Professor of Radiology, Division of Nuclear
Medicine, Department of Radiology, University
of Pennsylvania School of Medicine, Hospital
of the University of Pennsylvania, Philadelphia,
Pennsylvania

MANUEL BARDIÈS, PhD
UMR 1037 Inserm/UPS, Cancer Research
Center of Toulouse, Toulouse, France

SUSHIL BERIWAL, MD
Department of Radiation Oncology, University
of Pittsburgh Cancer Institute, Pittsburgh,
Pennsylvania

FRANÇOISE BONICHON, MD, MSc
Department of Nuclear Medicine, Institut
Bergonié, Bordeaux, France

BEN BOURSI, MD
Department of Gastroenterology, University of
Pennsylvania, Philadelphia, Pennsylvania

XAVIER BUY, MD
Department of Interventional Radiology,
Institut Bergonié, Bordeaux, France

PAOLO CASTELLUCCI, MD
Service of Nuclear Medicine,
S.Orsola-Malpighi Hospital, University of
Bologna, Bologna, Italy

FRANCESCO CECI, MD
Service of Nuclear Medicine,
S.Orsola-Malpighi Hospital, University of
Bologna, Bologna, Italy

STEFANO FANTI, MD
Service of Nuclear Medicine,
S.Orsola-Malpighi Hospital, University of
Bologna, Bologna, Italy

AFSHIN GANGI, MD, PhD
Non-Vascular IR Department, University
Hospital of Strasbourg, Strasbourg, France

PHILIPPE GARRIGUE, PharmD
Department of Radiopharmacy, La
Timone University Hospital, Aix-Marseille
University, Marseille, France

BEANT S. GILL, MD
Department of Radiation Oncology, University of Pittsburgh Cancer Institute, Pittsburgh, Pennsylvania

YANN GODBERT, MD
Department of Nuclear Medicine, Institut Bergonié, Bordeaux, France

TIZIANO GRAZIANI, MD
Service of Nuclear Medicine, S.Orsola-Malpighi Hospital, University of Bologna, Bologna, Italy

MICHAEL S. HOFMAN, MBBS, FRACP
Physician in Nuclear Medicine and Molecular Imaging; Associate Professor, Centre for Cancer Imaging, Peter MacCallum Cancer Centre, East Melbourne, Victoria, Australia; Department of Medicine, University of Melbourne, Melbourne, Victoria, Australia

SINA HOUSHMAND, MD
Department of Radiology, Hospital of the University of Pennsylvania, Philadelphia, Pennsylvania

RAKESH KUMAR, MD, PhD
Professor and Head, Diagnostic Nuclear Medicine Division, Department of Nuclear Medicine, All India Institute of Medical Sciences, New Delhi, India

STACEY McKENZIE, CNMT, RT (N), (CT)
Department of Radiation Oncology, University of Pittsburgh Cancer Institute, Pittsburgh, Pennsylvania

NAYELLI ORTEGA LÓPEZ, MD
Nuclear Medicine Physician, Department of Nuclear Medicine, Instituto Nacional de Cancerología; PET/CT Unit, Imagenus, Advanced Diagnostics in Healthcare, Mexico City, Mexico

KAREL PACAK, MD, PhD, DSc
Program in Reproductive and Adult Endocrinology, Eunice Kennedy Shriver National Institute of Child Health and Human Development (NICHD), National Institutes of Health, Bethesda, Maryland

SARAH S. PAI, MD
Department of Radiology, University of Pittsburgh Medical Center, Pittsburgh, Pennsylvania

JEAN PALUSSIÈRE, MD
Department of Interventional Radiology, Institut Bergonié, Bordeaux, France

DAVID A. PATTISON, MBBS, MPH, FRACP
Doctor, Centre for Cancer Imaging; Endocrinology Service, Peter MacCallum Cancer Centre, East Melbourne, Victoria, Australia

ALI SALAVATI, MD, MPH
Department of Radiology, Hospital of the University of Pennsylvania, Philadelphia, Pennsylvania; Department of Radiology, University of Minnesota, Minneapolis, Minnesota

RICCARDO SCHIAVINA, MD
Department of Urology, S.Orsola-Malpighi Hospital, University of Bologna, Bologna, Italy

PUNIT SHARMA, MD, FANMB
Department of Nuclear Medicine and PET/CT, Eastern Diagnostics India Ltd, Kolkata, India; Diagnostic Nuclear Medicine Division, Department of Nuclear Medicine, All India Institute of Medical Sciences, New Delhi, India

CHARLES B. SIMONE II, MD
Department of Radiation Oncology, University of Pennsylvania, Philadelphia, Pennsylvania

DAVID TAÏEB, MD, PhD
Department of Nuclear Medicine, La Timone University Hospital; European Center for Research in Medical Imaging, Aix-Marseille University; Marseille Cancerology Research Center, Inserm UMR1068, Institut Paoli-Calmettes, Marseille, France

Contents

This review provides practical guidance for clinicians involved in the management of endocrine malignancies, including endocrinologists, medical oncologists, surgeons and nuclear medicine specialists regarding the indications and use of 2-fluoro-2-deoxy-D-glucose F-18 (FDG) PET/computed tomography (CT), particularly with respect to targeted radionuclide therapy. Key principles of FDG PET/CT for radionuclide therapy are explored in detail using gastroenteropancreatic neuroendocrine tumors as a prototype endocrine malignancy. The relevant literature is reviewed, and practical application in this new and emerging field is highlighted with the use of case examples.

Neuroendocrine tumors (NETs) are associated with variable prognosis, with grade 1 and 2 NETs having more favorable outcomes than grade 3. Patients with gastroenteropancreatic (GEP)-NET need individualized interdisciplinary evaluations and treatment. New treatment options have become available with significant improvements in progression-free survival. Peptide receptor radionuclide therapy (PRRT) using ^{90}Y or ^{177}Lu-labeled somatostatin analogues (SSTa) has also shown promise in the treatment of advanced progressive NETs. ^{68}Ga-1,4,7,10-tetraazacyclodecane-1,4,7,10-tetraacetic acid (DOTA)-SSTa can be used as companion imaging agents to assist in radionuclide therapy selection. ^{68}Ga-DOTA-SSTa PET/computed tomography might also provide information for prognosis, tumor response assessment to PRRT, and internal dosimetry.

Choline PET/computed tomographic (CT) imaging represents the most diffused PET imaging techniques to investigate patients with prostate cancer (PCa). It may show the site of tumor recurrence in a single step examination, earlier than other conventional imaging techniques. In this context, the availability of a diagnostic test capable of differentiating between potentially curable local recurrence and metastatic disease implying palliative approaches may play an important role in those patients in whom targeted therapies could be performed according to choline PET/CT results. This review analyzes the value of choline PET/CT imaging in the evaluation of treatment of patients with PCa.

Targeted therapy is gaining prominence in the management of different cancers. Given different mechanism of action compared with traditional chemoradiotherapy, selection of patients for targeted therapy and monitoring response to these agents is difficult with conventional imaging. Various new PET radiopharmaceuticals have been evaluated for molecular imaging of these targets to achieve specific patient selection and response monitoring. These PET/computed tomography (CT) agents target the cell surface receptors, hormone receptors, receptor tyrosine kinases, or angiogenesis components. This article reviews the established and potential role of PET/CT with new radiopharmaceuticals for guiding targeted therapy.

Transarterial chemoembolization is a minimally invasive procedure that deprives the tumor of its blood supply, and is especially used for the treatment of unresectable hepatocellular carcinoma. Metabolic evaluation of interventional therapies such as transarterial chemoembolization in hepatocellular carcinoma is proving to be a valuable tool in choosing therapies that are better targeted to patients, especially because of its likely contribution in predicting treatment response in unresectable lesions after these therapies.

Thermal ablation (radiofrequency, microwave, cryosurgery, laser interstitial thermal therapy) is being used more frequently as a local treatment of secondary but also primary cancers and benign lesions. It has a low morbidity and is repeatable. The problem is that computed tomographic scan has limits, and RECIST criteria are not applicable. The objective of this article is to summarize the usefulness and pitfalls of PET/computed tomography in detecting a relapse after thermal ablation as soon as possible.

PET imaging has contributed substantially in oncology by allowing improved clinical staging and guiding appropriate cancer management. Integration with radiotherapy planning via PET/computed tomography (CT) simulation enables improved target delineation, which is paramount for conformal radiotherapy techniques. This article reviews the present literature regarding implications of PET/CT for radiotherapy planning and management.

One of the most important aspects of cancer treatment is radiation therapy, which is used for a wide range of malignancies. However, this treatment modality has side effects that impose the patient to increased risks of mortality and morbidity. Total dose, fraction size, and duration of radiation therapy are among the factors contributing to toxicities. In recent decades, fluorodeoxyglucose (FDG)-PET/computed tomography (CT) has been extensively used for diagnosis, prognostication, response to treatment assessment, and management of cancers and is currently a standard modality for many cancers. This article discusses the role of PET/CT, and especially FDG-PET/CT, in radiotherapy complications.

PET CLINICS

RELATED INTEREST

Radiologic Clinics, September 2015 (Vol. 53, Issue 5)
Oncology Imaging and Intervention in the Abdomen
Robert J. Lewandowski and Matthew S. Davenport, *Editors*
Available at: http://www.radiologic.theclinics.com

THE CLINICS ARE AVAILABLE ONLINE!
Access your subscription at:
www.theclinics.com

PROGRAM OBJECTIVE

The goal of the *PET Clinics* is to keep practicing radiologists and radiology residents up to date with current clinical practice in positron emission tomography by providing timely articles reviewing the state of the art in patient care.

TARGET AUDIENCE

Practicing radiologists, radiology residents, and other health care professionals who provide patient care utilizing radiologic findings.

LEARNING OBJECTIVES

Upon completion of this activity, participants will be able to:
1. Review the use of PET imaging in radiotherapy treatment planning.
2. Discuss applications of PET/CT in targeted treatments and therapies for malignancies.
3. Recognize the process and goals of targeted radionuclide therapy for gastroenteropancreatic neuroendocrine tumors.

ACCREDITATION

The Elsevier Office of Continuing Medical Education (EOCME) is accredited by the Accreditation Council for Continuing Medical Education (ACCME) to provide continuing medical education for physicians.

The EOCME designates this enduring material for a maximum of 15 *AMA PRA Category 1 Credit*(s)™. Physicians should claim only the credit commensurate with the extent of their participation in the activity.

All other health care professionals requesting continuing education credit for this enduring material will be issued a certificate of participation.

DISCLOSURE OF CONFLICTS OF INTEREST

The EOCME assesses conflict of interest with its instructors, faculty, planners, and other individuals who are in a position to control the content of CME activities. All relevant conflicts of interest that are identified are thoroughly vetted by EOCME for fair balance, scientific objectivity, and patient care recommendations. EOCME is committed to providing its learners with CME activities that promote improvements or quality in healthcare and not a specific proprietary business or a commercial interest.

The planning committee, staff, authors and editors listed below have identified no financial relationships or relationships to products or devices they or their spouse/life partner have with commercial interest related to the content of this CME activity:

Ahmad Esmaeel Abdullah, MD; Abass Alavi, MD, PhD (Hon), Dsc (Hon); Manuel Bardiès, PhD; Sushil Beriwal, MD; Françoise Bonichon, MD, MSc; Ben Boursi, MD; Xavier Buy, MD; Paolo Castellucci, MD; Francesco Ceci, MD; Anjali Fortna; Afshin Gangi, MD, PhD; Philippe Garrigue, PharmD; Beant S. Gill, MD; Yann Godbert, MD; Tiziano Graziani, MD; Michael S. Hofman, MBBS, FRACP; Sina Houshmand, MD; Rakesh Kumar, MD, PhD; Stacey McKenzie, CNMT, RT (N), (CT); Nayelli Ortega López, MD; Mahalakshmi Narayanan; Karel Pacak, MD, PhD, DSc; Sarah S. Pai, MD; Jean Palussière, MD; David A. Pattison, MBBS, MPH, FRACP; Ali Salavati, MD, MPH; Erin Scheckenbach; Riccardo Schiavina, MD; Punit Sharma, MD, FANMB; Charles B. Simone II, MD; David Taïeb, MD, PhD; John Vassallo.

The planning committee, staff, authors and editors listed below have identified financial relationships or relationships to products or devices they or their spouse/life partner have with commercial interest related to the content of this CME activity:

Stefano Fanti, MD is on the speakers' bureau for Blue Earth Diagnostics Limited and General Electric Company, and is a consultant/advisor for Janssen Global Services, LLC: Pharmaceutical Companies of Johnson & Johnson.

UNAPPROVED/OFF-LABEL USE DISCLOSURE

The EOCME requires CME faculty to disclose to the participants:
1. When products or procedures being discussed are off-label, unlabelled, experimental, and/or investigational (not US Food and Drug Administration [FDA] approved); and
2. Any limitations on the information presented, such as data that are preliminary or that represent ongoing research, interim analyses, and/or unsupported opinions. Faculty may discuss information about pharmaceutical agents that is outside of FDA-approved labelling. This information is intended solely for CME and is not intended to promote off-label use of these medications. If you have any questions, contact the medical affairs department of the manufacturer for the most recent prescribing information.

TO ENROLL

To enroll in the *PET Clinics* Continuing Medical Education program, call customer service at 1-800-654-2452 or sign up online at http://www.theclinics.com/home/cme. The CME program is available to subscribers for an additional annual fee of USD $235.

METHOD OF PARTICIPATION

In order to claim credit, participants must complete the following:

1. Complete enrolment as indicated above.
2. Read the activity.
3. Complete the CME Test and Evaluation. Participants must achieve a score of 70% on the test. All CME Tests and Evaluations must be completed online.

CME INQUIRIES/SPECIAL NEEDS

For all CME inquiries or special needs, please contact elsevierCME@elsevier.com.

Preface
PET/Computed Tomography-based Intervention

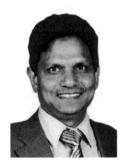

Rakesh Kumar, MD, PhD
Editor

PET/computed tomography (CT) plays an important role in staging, treatment response evaluation, restaging, and prognostication of various cancers. The synergistic use of structural and functional imaging provides excellent information regarding the disease. Changes at the molecular and cellular levels can be imaged effectively through specific radiopharmaceuticals using PET/CT for evaluating the effectiveness of chosen clinical treatment plans. Therefore, PET/CT allows the individualization of treatment for patients with cancer. These targeted therapies are aimed at various receptors, enzymes, or pathways, and hence, are less toxic and more specific than conventional chemoradiotherapies. Molecular imaging with PET can visualize such targets or biochemical processes and/or their dysfunction using specific radiopharmaceuticals. These radiopharmaceuticals help in identification of the presence or absence of various targets in cancer cells for directed therapy, and thus, can help in determining the suitability of patients for targeted therapy. Various such radiopharmaceuticals have been developed and explored in the last decade or so of which imaging of the somatostatin receptor using gallium-68-1,4,7,10-tetraazacyclododecane-1,4,7,10-tetraacetic acid (68Ga-DOTA) peptides has gained considerable popularity. Other popular molecular imaging agents used for targeted therapy include 68Ga-prostate-specific membrane antigen (PSMA) PET/CT in patients with prostate cancer (PCa), and 16α-[18F]-fluoro-17β-estradiol (18F-FES) PET/CT in patients with breast cancer. Various PET radiopharmaceuticals directed against tyrosine kinase

receptor, such as 64Cu/89Zr-trastuzumab63 for HER2 and64Cu/86Y/89Zr-cetuximab and 64Cu/86Y/89Zrpanitumumab for EGFR, are also gaining popularity as molecular imaging probes for individualized targeted therapies.

This issue of *PET Clinics* has been prepared in the hope that it will help in the understanding of the role of PET/CT as a molecular imaging modality that can help in determining the suitability of patients for targeted therapy with different agents and the role of PET/CT in selecting patients with appropriate treatment and response.

Drs Pattison and Hofman describe the role of 2-fluoro-2-deoxy-D-glucose F18 (FDG) PET/CT in targeted radionuclide therapy of endocrine malignancies. FDG-PET/CT is the most powerful prognostic indicator in common endocrine malignancies (including gastroenteropancreatic neuroendocrine tumors [NETs] and differentiated thyroid cancer) facilitating risk stratification and optimization of personalized therapy. In these malignancies, increased FDG uptake represents dedifferentiated disease. However, in endocrine malignancy, intense FDG uptake does not always indicate dedifferentiated disease. In pseudohypoxic pheochromocytoma and paraganglioma and oncocytic thyroid tumors, intense FDG avidity is noted due to intrinsic mitochondrial dysfunction.

Drs Taïeb, Garrigue, Bardiès, Esmaeel, and Pacak show various application and dosimetric requirements for 68Ga-labeled somatostatin analogues in targeted radionuclide therapy for gastroenteropancreatic neuroendocrine tumors. PET/CT using gallium-68–labeled SSTa is a popular

http://dx.doi.org/10.1016/j.cpet.2015.07.001
1556-8598/15/$ – see front matter © 2015 Published by Elsevier Inc.

pet.theclinics.com

PET-based theranostic approach that provides prognostic information, selecting good candidates for peptide receptor radionuclide therapy (PRRT) and enabling tumor response assessment for PRRT. PRRT using 177Lu-labeled SSTa has also shown promise in the treatment of advanced progressive grade 1 and 2 NETs. Theranostics of gastroenteropancreatic NETs based on 68Ga-labeled SSTa PET imaging and targeted therapy applying PRRT with 90Y-labeled and/or 177Lu-labeled SSTa have paved the way for personalized medicine.

Drs Ceci, Castellucci, Graziani, Schiavina, and Fanti review the role of PET/CT in the individualization of the treatment of PCa. Choline is a promising PET agent for imaging of PCa. PET/CT using choline in patients with relapsed PCa show the site of tumor recurrence earlier than other conventional imaging techniques. It also helps to guide personalized therapies in patients with oligometastatic disease. The addition of choline PET/CT as a diagnostic modality in patients with PCa may affect significantly treatment strategies and patient management.

Drs Sharma, Kumar, and Alavi summarize the individualized targeted therapies aimed at various receptors, enzymes, or pathways. Various such radiopharmaceuticals have been developed and explored in the last decade or so, including imaging of the somatostatin receptor using 68Ga-DOTA peptides, 68Ga-PSMA PET/CT in the patients with PCa, and 18F-FES PET/CT in patients with breast cancer. Various PET radiopharmaceuticals directed against tyrosine kinase receptor, such as 64Cu/89Zr-trastuzumab63 for HER2, and64Cu/86Y/89Zr-cetuximab and 64Cu/86Y/89Zrpanitumumab for EGFR, are also gaining popularity as molecular imaging probes for individualized targeted therapies.

Dr López describes the role of PET/CT in the evaluation of transarterial chemoembolization, which is a minimally invasive procedure that deprives the tumor of its blood supply and is especially used for the treatment of unresectable hepatocellular carcinoma. During chemoembolization, PET/CT is a useful tool for early recognition of incomplete tumor destruction. It also detects recurrence earlier than the conventional imaging modalities. Thus, FDG-PET/CT is one of the most useful imaging modalities in patients undergoing transarterial chemoembolization.

Drs Bonichon, Godbert, Gangi, Buy, and Palussière share their experience using PET/CT in thermoablation techniques. Thermal ablation is more frequently used in oncology for primary and secondary cancer but is also used to destroy benign tumors. PET/CT plays an important role in the follow-up to detect residual viable tissue and early detection of a relapse that can be re-treated by thermal ablation or other means. Postablation aspects have to be well known by the specialist in charge of image interpretation. All studies done based on thermal ablation conclude that PET/CT is a useful tool for early recognition of incomplete tumor destruction after thermal ablation.

Drs Gill, Pai, McKenzie, and Beriwal review the utility of PET/CT for radiotherapy treatment planning. Development and accessibility of PET/CT have considerably changed patient management in oncology, allowing for more accurate clinical staging and target delineation for radiotherapy. Integration with radiotherapy planning, either at the time of simulation or with image fusion, has enabled adaptive planning and has become an additive tool to ensure accurate target delineation. Considerable work has been completed to demonstrate the value of PET/CT for radiotherapy planning, showing that in several malignancies like head and neck carcinoma, lung carcinoma, and gynecologic malignancy, this approach can lead to more accurate tumor targeting and can alter radiotherapy plans significantly. Continued research is needed to establish uniform contouring guidelines and evaluate the clinical impact of PET-based planning, with regard to both toxicity and disease control.

Drs Houshmand, Boursi, Salavati, Simone, and Alavi describe the FDG-PET/CT in the assessment and prediction of radiation therapy–related complications. Radiation pneumonitis is a life-threatening acute and subacute complication of radiation therapy happening in 4% to 30% of patients and manifesting 1 to 6 months after radiation. Detection of radiation pneumonitis, sometimes challenged by using other clinical criteria, might be aided by accurate and quantitative PET parameters before or after RT. FDG-PET/CT has also been shown to be feasible for the assessment of cardiovascular adverse events, such as vascular inflammation and cardiomyopathies. PET/CT is a valuable imaging modality to detect the effects of RT on the human body and the evolution of the short-term and long-term complications of RT and chemotherapy.

Rakesh Kumar, MD, PhD
Diagnostic Nuclear Medicine Division
Department of Nuclear Medicine
All India Institute of Medical Sciences
Ansari Nagar
New Delhi 110029, India

E-mail address:
rkphulia@hotmail.com

Role of Fluorodeoxyglucose PET/Computed Tomography in Targeted Radionuclide Therapy for Endocrine Malignancies

David A. Pattison, MBBS, MPH, FRACP[a,b],
Michael S. Hofman, MBBS, FRACP[a,c,*]

KEYWORDS

- FDG PET/CT • Radionuclide therapy • Peptide receptor radionuclide therapy
- Neuroendocrine tumor • Thyroid cancer

KEY POINTS

- Endocrine malignancies demonstrate a spectrum of clinical behaviors from benign, well-differentiated hormone-producing tumors to malignant, poorly differentiated carcinomas.
- A single, unselected biopsy is not representative of overall disease grade because of tumor heterogeneity, with different tumor phenotypes at different sites.
- 2-Fluoro-2-deoxy-D-glucose F-18 (FDG) PET/computed tomography (CT) is the most powerful prognostic indicator in common endocrine malignancies (including gastroenteropancreatic [GEP] neuroendocrine tumors [NETs] and differentiated thyroid cancer [DTC]) facilitating risk stratification and optimization of personalized therapy.
- The flip-flop phenomenon of increasing FDG uptake with increasing tumor dedifferentiation (and loss of molecular imaging targets such as somatostatin receptor [SSTR] expression or Na/iodide symporter) is well described in endocrine malignancies.
- Intense FDG uptake does not always indicate dedifferentiated disease, with pseudohypoxic pheochromocytoma and paraganglioma (PPGL) and oncocytic thyroid tumors characterized by intense FDG avidity due to intrinsic mitochondrial dysfunction in both benign and malignant disease alike.

INTRODUCTION

The role of FDG PET/CT in the management of endocrine malignancies has evolved over the last 15 years with increasing clinical experience and greater understanding of the mechanism of disease-specific uptake and its implications. The utility of FDG PET/CT as a diagnostic test in unselected populations of these endocrine malignancies was initially underestimated given the frequent low intrinsic metabolic activity and lack of tumor specificity in most of these tumors, particularly in an era of targeted imaging agents, including SSTR and metaiodobenzylguanidine

The authors have nothing to disclose.
[a] Centre for Cancer Imaging, Peter MacCallum Cancer Centre, East Melbourne, Victoria, Australia; [b] Endocrinology Service, Peter MacCallum Cancer Centre, East Melbourne, Victoria, Australia; [c] Department of Medicine, University of Melbourne, Melbourne, Victoria, Australia
* Corresponding author. Centre for Cancer Imaging, Peter MacCallum Cancer Centre, 7 St Andrew's Place, East Melbourne, Victoria 3000, Australia.
E-mail address: Michael.Hofman@petermac.org

PET Clin 10 (2015) 461–476
http://dx.doi.org/10.1016/j.cpet.2015.05.005
1556-8598/15/$ – see front matter © 2015 Elsevier Inc. All rights reserved.

(MIBG) imaging. Initially, the role of FDG in the imaging of NETs (like much of oncology) was considered limited to a diagnostic test for defining the extent of disease and was deemed only to be of value if other molecular imaging (eg, SSTR scintigraphy) findings were negative.[1] However, increasing experience with FDG has also facilitated greater understanding of the appropriate clinical indications for FDG imaging in these tumor types to maximize management impact.

Endocrine malignancies often demonstrate a broad spectrum of clinical behavior ranging from benign, well-differentiated tumors that may produce a variety of hormones to malignant, poorly differentiated carcinomas. Consequently, there is a risk of overtreating those tumors at the benign end of the spectrum or underestimating the rapidity of progression in those with a more aggressive phenotype.

Risk stratification and treatment selection is critically important to the delivery of targeted, appropriate personalized therapy.[2] There are significant limitations with traditional prognostic markers including disease staging systems and histopathologic markers. In the evolving literature, the degree of glycolytic metabolic activity as reflected by FDG uptake intensity consistently outperforms these in many endocrine malignancies. In this context, a negative FDG PET/CT scan result in a patient with known metastatic disease indicates something fundamental about the indolent biology of the tumor and potentially indicates that a period of observation to better define the disease natural history may be appropriate, rather than representing a poor diagnostic test with low sensitivity. However, the patient with extensive dedifferentiated FDG-avid disease warrants a more aggressive treatment approach given the poorer prognosis.

In addition to this broad variability in biology between patients, there is an increasing recognition of the importance of tumor heterogeneity within the same patient.[3] The use of FDG PET/CT can provide useful information to guide biopsy and facilitate appropriate treatment targeted to the most metabolically active and aggressive site of disease. Assessment of concordance between a theranostic radionuclide and sites of dedifferentiated disease is critical to predict and optimize a favorable treatment response.

MECHANISM OF FLUORODEOXYGLUCOSE UPTAKE IN ENDOCRINE MALIGNANCY

The enhanced uptake of glucose by tumor cells relative to normal cells is the hallmark of in vivo cancer imaging with FDG PET/CT. In contrast to normal differentiated cells and well-differentiated endocrine tumors reliant on mitochondrial oxidative phosphorylation to generate the energy needed for cellular processes, poorly differentiated cancer cells depend on the inefficient mechanism of aerobic glycolysis, termed the Warburg effect,[4] to fuel their metabolic needs. ^{18}F-FDG is a glucose analogue taken up by cancer cells via facilitative transport by glucose transporters (GLUT) and phosphorylated by intracellular hexokinase yielding ^{18}F-FDG-6-phosphate, which (unlike glucose-6-phosphate) cannot be metabolized further in the glycolytic pathway or exit the cell. The FDG uptake of any cell is determined by the expression of GLUTs, hexokinase, and tumoral blood flow for delivery of tracer.

Numerous studies have demonstrated a correlation between increasing FDG avidity and poor prognosis in GEP-NETs, medullary thyroid cancer (MTC), PPGL, and DTC. A flip-flop phenomenon is also well described, whereby well-differentiated thyroid carcinoma retains activity of the sodium iodide symporter and iodine avidity (with low glucose requirements similar to normal cells), with subsequent loss of iodine avidity and resulting increased FDG avidity in sites of poorly differentiated disease.[5] This phenomenon has also been long recognized in NETs, MTCs,[1] and PPGL. However, it is important to recognize that this dedifferentiation process represents a spectrum rather than a binary switch, with a substantial proportion of patients demonstrating features of both a well-differentiated phenotype (SSTR expression or Na/iodide symporter activity) and enhanced glycolytic activity. For example, a recent analysis of distant metastatic lesions in DTC identified radioiodine uptake in 33% (60 of 181) of FDG avid lesions, potentially amenable to radionuclide therapy.[6]

It is also important to note that the driver of increased glycolytic metabolism varies between tumor subtypes, with 2 particular exceptions of critical importance. PPGL susceptibility genes are divided into 2 groups, with the uptake on FDG PET/CT imaging of PPGLs observed in cluster 1, which demonstrates increased expression of genes associated with angiogenesis and hypoxia (pseudohypoxic cluster) comprising succinate dehydrogenase (SDH) complex units and assembly factor 2 (SDHA/B/C/D/AF2) in addition to von-Hippel-Lindau (VHL). Cluster 2 includes RET (REarranged during Transfection), neurofibromatosis 1 (NF1), myc-associated factor X (MAX), and transmembrane protein 127 (TMEM127) susceptibility genes involved in kinase signaling pathways. Mutations in cluster 1 susceptibility genes lead to constitutive activation of hypoxia-inducible factors (HIFs) regardless of oxygen levels, with resultant inhibition of oxidative phosphorylation and induction of glycolytic pathways consistent with the Warburg effect. The resultant intense FDG uptake occurs despite a benign differentiated phenotype.[7] A study by van Berkel and colleagues[8] indicated that the activation of aerobic glycolysis in SDHx-related PPGLs is associated with increased FDG accumulation due to accelerated glucose phosphorylation by hexokinases (HK-2 and HK-3) rather than increased expression of glucose transporters (GLUT-1 and GLUT-3).

Oncocytic tumors are another group for which intense FDG avidity represents inherent constitutive activation of glycolytic pathways rather than a poorly differentiated phenotype (**Fig. 1**). This group includes Hürthle cell neoplasm in the thyroid,[9,10] Warthin tumors in the salivary glands (typically the parotid), and oncocytomas arising in the kidney and other organs. These tumors are defined histologically by the presence of a granular cytoplasm due to mitochondrial hyperproliferation. Loss of the mitochondrial respiratory chain complex I has been shown to be a molecular marker of the oncocytic phenotype,[11] leading to mitochondrial dysfunction, inhibition of oxidative phosphorylation, and upregulation of glycolytic metabolism in a pattern similar to SDH (complex II) mutations.

ROLE OF FLUORODEOXYGLUCOSE PET/COMPUTED TOMOGRAPHY IN THE MANAGEMENT OF GASTROENTEROPANCREATIC NEUROENDOCRINE TUMORS

Molecular imaging is transforming management of patients with NETs by enabling powerful disease characterization. This improved definition of disease phenotype is pivotal in personalizing care and assessing the treatment most likely to beneficial for an individual, including suitability for targeted treatment with peptide receptor radionuclide therapy (PRRT). Conventional diagnostic paradigms in patients with metastatic disease rely on histopathologic assessment from a single site, usually the site most amenable to surgical or percutaneous biopsy. It is increasingly recognized, however, that a single biopsy cannot be considered representative owing to tumor heterogeneity with different phenotypes of disease possible at various sites.[3] NETs exhibit marked

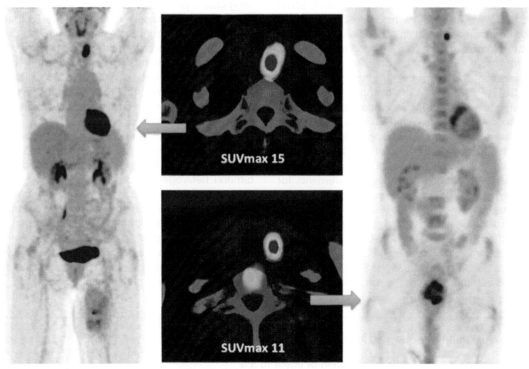

Fig. 1. Intensely FDG-avid benign Hürthle cell adenomas. FDG PET maximum intensity projections and fused axial FDG PET/CT slices through the thyroid demonstrate intense FDG uptake (maximum standardized uptake value 15 and 11) in histopathologically confirmed benign Hürthle cell adenomas. FDG uptake in Hürthle cell neoplasms (benign and malignant) is not a marker of dedifferentiation but represents a specific defect in oxidative phosphorylation leading to markedly increased glucose utilization via aerobic glycolysis.

variation in tumor biology from highly indolent well-differentiated to highly aggressive poorly differentiated phenotypes making them a tumor type in which accurate characterization is pivotal in determining the optimal management strategy (**Box 1**).

FLUORODEOXYGLUCOSE VERSUS SOMATOSTATIN RECEPTOR PET/CT

According to their degree of differentiation, NETs variably express SSTRs on their cell surface. This feature is used for both imaging and therapy using radiolabeled somatostatin analogues. Imaging is primarily performed with ^{111}In single-photon emission computed tomography (SPECT)/CT or ^{68}Ga PET/CT, whereas the beta emitters ^{177}Lu and ^{90}Y are used for radionuclide therapy. [68]Ga SSTR PET/CT imaging has emerged as the new gold standard for imaging NETs, with extraordinary sensitivity and specificity compared with conventional imaging[12] with consequent high management impact.[13] Although many diagnostic imaging studies focus on accuracy as assessed with sensitivity and specificity, an area of paradigm change is the use of imaging to characterize disease.[14]

FDG PET/CT plays a complementary and important role to tumor-specific imaging with SSTR PET/CT. We and others have described a flip-flop phenomenon in which well-differentiated sites that resemble the normal neuroendocrine tissue from which the tumor arose retain high SSTR expression and consequently have high uptake on SSTR PET/CT.[14–16] The histopathologic correlate is a low level of Ki,67, a marker of cellular proliferation, and tumors with Ki,67 less than 2% are classified as grade 1 according to the European Neuroendocrine Tumor Society (ENETS) grading system.[17] Commensurate with their low proliferative rate such tumors have low requirements for glycolytic metabolism and consequently no or minimal uptake on FDG PET/CT. Conversely, NETs at the other end of the spectrum with Ki,67 more than 20% are defined as ENETS grade 3 tumors and invariably have high FDG uptake. These tumor sites typically have lower SSTR expression, with lower-intensity uptake on SSTR PET/CT.

However, a proportion of these tumors retain high uptake on both SSTR and FDG PET/CT, whereas the more aggressive NETs may lose or not express SSTR altogether (**Fig. 2**).

It is an oversimplification to describe the relationship of SSTR and FDG PET/CT as inverse, and understanding the reasons for NETs that do not conform to these simplicities is increasingly important to maximize the utility of molecular imaging for disease characterization. As depicted in **Fig. 3**, although rare, a small proportion of well-differentiated low-grade tumors may have high FDG or low SSTR uptake on PET/CT. The high FDG uptake in these NETs is not well understood and may relate to disorders in oxidative phosphorylation resulting in high glycolytic metabolism despite an indolent phenotype. This phenomenon has been best characterized with the pseudohypoxic cluster pheochromocytomas and is discussed later. The absence of SSTR uptake in a small proportion of indolent NETs simply reflects lack of SSTR expression, which, although characteristic of well-differentiated tumors, is not universal; for example, a proportion of benign insulinomas do not express SSTR. On the other end of the spectrum, a proportion of more aggressive NETs lack high FDG uptake despite a progressive phenotype. Evolving experience suggests that this is observed in some ENETS grade 2 tumors arising from the small bowel. This phenomenon is also not well understood but likely relates to use of metabolic pathways other than glycolytic metabolism (eg, glutamine[18]) for growth. In summary, it is important to interpret the FDG intensity in the context of both temporal change and histopathologic findings.

In some patients, there is marked intertumoral heterogeneity with varying phenotypes of tumor at different sites. The lack of ability to identify intertumoral heterogeneity with traditional diagnostic paradigms of anatomic imaging and random biopsy has been a serious flaw in oncology leading to incorrect selection of therapy. For example, for a patient with poorly differentiated disease in whom a random biopsy characterizes the disease as well differentiated, hormonal therapy may be started; only after subsequent recognition of

---

Box 1
Suggested indications for FDG PET/CT in NETs

- Patients with Ki,67 levels greater than or equal to 5%
- Patients with clinical or imaging findings of progressive disease within a 6-month period
- Patients with sites of disease identified on CT that do not have uptake on SSTR PET/CT and are of concern as sites of poorly differentiated disease

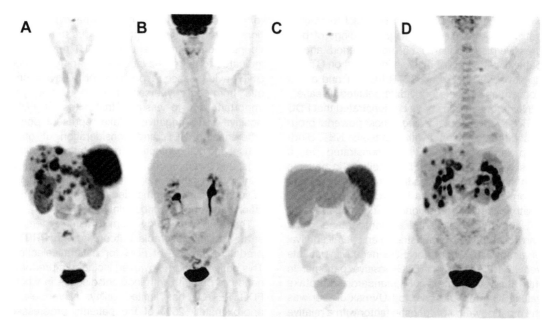

Fig. 2. Patterns of SSTR- and FDG-avid neuroendocrine tumors (NETs). Maximum intensity projection images of 2 patients with NETs and widespread hepatic metastases. (*A*) DOTATATE and (*B*) FDG PET/CT in the first patient demonstrate SSTR-positive FDG-negative phenotype, whereas (*C*) DOTATATE and (*D*) FDG PET/CT in the second patient demonstrate the opposite phenotype. The first patient (*left*) has an ENETS grade 1 (Ki,67 <1%) well-differentiated metastatic tumor, whereas the second patient (*right*) has a poorly differentiated ENETS grade 3 (Ki,67 = 70%) neuroendocrine carcinoma. The FDG PET/CTs provide powerful prognostic information in these patients.

disease progression is treatment redirected. The ability of molecular imaging to provide whole-body disease characterization is a key component of personalizing care in our NET multidisciplinary service.[19] Owing to the short half-life of ^{68}Ga, it is feasible to perform both SSTR and FDG PET/CT on the same day. In our current practice, we perform FDG PET/CT selectively in (1) patients

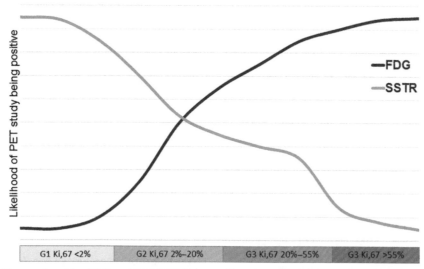

Fig. 3. Likelihood of positive SSTR and FDG PET/CT depending on proliferative rate in patients with neuroendocrine tumors. Most but not all patients with indolent well-differentiated tumors have SSTR-positive FDG-negative disease, whereas patients with aggressive poorly differentiated carcinomas have SSTR-negative FDG-positive disease. Patients in the middle of the spectrum have both SSTR- and FDG positivity. Patients under the green line are potential candidates for peptide receptor radionuclide therapy.

with Ki,67 level greater than or equal to 5%, (2) patients with clinical or imaging findings of progressive disease within a 6-month period, and (3) patients with sites of disease identified on CT that do not have uptake on SSTR PET/CT and are of concern as sites of poorly differentiated disease.

Numerous studies have demonstrated that FDG PET/CT represents the single most powerful prognostic tool in patients with metastatic NET. Binderup and colleagues[20] demonstrated in a prospective study that FDG positivity in patients with metastatic NET was the strongest prognosticator for survival with a hazard radio of 10.3 of death, exceeding traditional markers such as Ki-67, chromogranin-A, and anatomic stage. Bahri and colleagues[21] demonstrated an overall survival of almost 10 years for FDG-negative patients versus 1.25 years for FDG-positive patients. In this study, the maximum standardized uptake value (SUVmax) of tumor to SUVmax of liver was the most powerful prognostic factor with a relative risk for death of 26.8 compared with 3.5 for Ki,67. Using the tumor to liver ratio, Ezziddin and colleagues[22] similarly demonstrated powerful risk stratification for survival with FDG PET/CT. In this study, patients were divided into 3 metabolic grades using cutoff of less than or equal to 1, greater than 1 to 2.3, and greater than 2.3. Patients with a high metabolic grade had inferior survival, and FDG PET/CT was the most powerful predictor in multivariate analysis.

Using Fluorodeoxyglucose for Assessment of Suitability of Peptide Receptor Radionuclide Therapy

FDG PET/CT forms a pivotal component of assessment of suitability for PRRT by enabling assessment of whether all sites of disease can be targeted with PRRT. Patients with FDG-positive SSTR-positive phenotype are suitable for PRRT, whereas patients with FDG-positive SSTR-negative phenotypes are generally not suitable. Therefore, FDG positivity is not by itself a contraindication to PRRT. In our experience, such patients with an aggressive phenotype may have the most spectacular responses to PRRT. Patients with FDG-positive disease are only excluded if there are sites of FDG-avid disease that do not demonstrate spatially concordant uptake on SSTR SPECT/CT (**Fig. 4**). Sites of FDG-positive, SSTR-negative disease cannot be targeted with PRRT but constitute the sites of most aggressive disease that are most likely to progress; treating sites of indolent disease in this context is usually of no benefit from an oncologic perspective. However, if treatment is indicated

for relief of symptoms from hormonal hypersecretion (eg, refractory hypoglycemia due to metastatic insulinoma), treatment with PRRT may still be indicated to target the indolent/well-differentiated SSTR-avid disease responsible for the symptomatic hormonal hypersecretion. It is, however, important not to assume that sites of FDG-positive SSTR-negative uptake represent poorly differentiated NET, and consideration of other causes including infection, incidental benign findings, and synchronous nonneuroendocrine malignancy needs to be considered. Directed biopsy of such sites is recommended for histologic correlation when there is uncertainty.

The landmark study from Erasmus demonstrated highly favorable outcomes with PRRT[23] predating the use of FDG for patient selection. This patient cohort, however, included a predominance of patients with indolent disease in whom FDG PET/CT has limited utility. Nevertheless, approximately 20% of the patients progressed despite PRRT. We believe that a proportion of these patients who primarily progressed had sites of FDG-positive SSTR-negative disease at baseline, and this failure may have therefore been predicted had FDG been performed. In our experience, when using FDG to exclude patients with spatially discordant disease that can be targeted, the incidence of primary progression is much lower.[24]

Many other treatment options remain for patients with FDG-positive SSTR-negative sites of disease that are not candidates for PRRT, including systemic chemotherapy, newer agents such as everolimus and sunitinib, liver-directed therapies, or surgery. If sites of FDG-positive SSTR-negative can be eradicated, they may become suitable for PRRT (**Fig. 5**). Our group and others combine PRRT with radiosensitizing chemotherapy such as 5-fluorouracil or capecitabine. Although these single-agent radiosensitizing regimens have limited utility in targeting sites of FDG-positive STTR-negative disease, newer more active regimens such as capecitabine and temozolomide (CAPTEM) may be effective.[25] Thus, patients deemed unsuitable for PRRT by virtue of some sites that are FDG-positive SSTR-negative may be suitable for and benefit from the combination of PRRT and CAPTEM or other emerging combination therapies.

Using Fluorodeoxyglucose for Response Assessment After Peptide Receptor Radionuclide Therapy

Traditional response assessment relies on the measurement of changes in the size of the lesions.

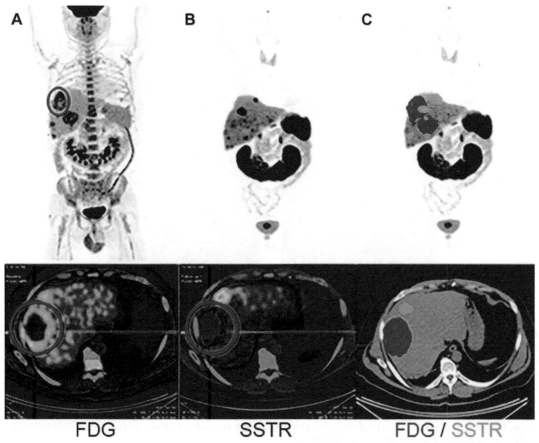

Fig. 4. Heterogeneous disease phenotypes at different sites in a patient with metastatic neuroendocrine tumor. Maximum intensity projection (MIP) image of (*A*) FDG and (*B*) DOTATATE PET/CT in a patient with metastatic NET with some sites of disease that are FDG-positive SSTR-negative (*red circle*). Other sites of disease are either FDG positive SSTR positive or FDG negative SSTR negative. MIP image (*C*) highlights sites of disease that can be targeted with peptide receptor radionuclide therapy in green, whereas 2 dominant sites of FDG-positive disease (*red*) are not SSTR avid and cannot be targeted.

Many studies use the Response Evaluation Criteria in Solid Tumors (RECIST) to dichotomize response.[26] Progressive disease is defined by an increase in the sum of the diameters of target lesions size by greater than 20%, whereas a partial response is defined by a decrease of 30%. With PRRT, high doses of radiation are delivered to tumors, which can result in cystic necrosis and consequent increase in the size of the tumor masses before shrinkage is subsequently observed. In patients with FDG-avid disease at baseline, we routinely incorporate restaging with FDG PET/CT 3 months postcompletion of PRRT. Relying on anatomic assessment with CT or MR imaging alone, especially when performed during or within several months of PRRT, misclassifies some patients who are responding as progressive disease.

Achieving a complete metabolic response after PRRT in patients with FDG-avid disease at baseline is a powerful prognostic factor, even in the presence of residual anatomic or SSTR-avid disease. The effects of PRRT can continue for many months after PRRT, and some patients subsequently achieve a complete metabolic response after having only a partial metabolic response at 3 months. In our cohort of 52 patients treated with ^{177}Lu DOTA-Octreotate (DOTATATE) (LuTate) in combination with radiosensitizing 5-fluorouracil, progression-free survival was 17 months in patients who achieved a partial metabolic response, although it was not reached in patients who achieved a complete metabolic response ($P<.001$) (median follow-up period of 36 months). Severi and colleagues[27] also demonstrated prognostic utility of FDG after PRRT in patients treated with stand-alone LuTate.

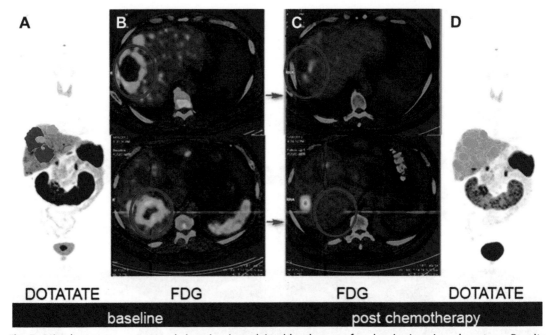

A DOTATATE **B** FDG **C** FDG **D** DOTATATE

baseline   post chemotherapy

Fig. 5. Mixed response on anatomic imaging is explained by change of molecular imaging phenotype. Despite some sites of SSTR-positive disease, this patient had 2 sites of FDG-positive SSTR-negative sites, which could not be potentially targeted with PRRT [(A) DOTATATE maximum intensity projection [MIP] with sites of discordant FDG-positive/SSTR-negative disease highlighted in red and sites of SSTR-positive disease in green, (B) baseline FDG PET/CT with red circle around discordant sites]. After 6 cycles of carboplatin-cisplatin chemotherapy, there was (C) a complete response in the 2 FDG-positive/SSTR-negative sites of disease, combined with marked decrease in size. Sites of SSTR-positive disease, however, had progressed, resulting in a mixed response on anatomic imaging alone. After chemotherapy, all sites of demonstrable disease are amenable to targeting with PRRT [(D) DOTATATE MIP after chemotherapy with lesions highlighted].

ROLE OF FLUORODEOXYGLUCOSE PET/ COMPUTED TOMOGRAPHY IN THE MANAGEMENT OF DIFFERENTIATED THYROID CANCER

Perioperative FDG PET/CT is not justified in most cases of DTC given the excellent long-term prognosis, indolent nature, and infrequent presentation with distant metastatic disease.[28] However, it has an important role in baseline or postoperative staging of more aggressive subtypes of thyroid cancer (tall cell, poorly differentiated, and anaplastic),[29] which are more likely to demonstrate FDG avidity because of dedifferentiation and have occult distant metastatic disease (**Box 2**). As previously discussed, Hürthle cell carcinoma demonstrates high intrinsic glycolytic activity due to a mitochondrial defect in oxidative phosphorylation, resulting in excellent accuracy for identification of disease. Although Hürthle cell carcinoma has a less favorable prognosis than

---

Box 2
Indications for FDG PET/CT in thyroid cancer

- Staging of patients with higher risk of metastatic disease
  - Hürthle cell and aggressive subtypes of thyroid cancer (tall cell, poorly differentiated subtypes)
- Assessment of patients with metastatic disease
  - Theranostic tool to determine suitability for radionuclide therapy by excluding spatially discordant iodine-negative/FDG-positive disease
  - Prognostic tool to identify sites of disease at the highest risk for rapid disease progression and also risk of patient mortality
- Assessment of increasing thyroglobulin level with negative radioiodine imaging
- Evaluation of posttreatment response

differentiated thyroid carcinoma, the high FDG uptake is a metabolic signature of this tumor (evident in benign adenomas and carcinomas alike) and not necessarily a marker of dedifferentiated disease. Pryma and colleagues[30] report a series of 44 patients describing sensitivity of 95.8% and specificity of 95%, recommending it as an important baseline postoperative investigation and if there is clinical or biochemical suspicion of recurrent/metastatic disease.

Prognostic Value of Fluorodeoxyglucose in Differentiated Thyroid Cancer

FDG PET/CT plays an important role in facilitating delivery of personalized management of DTC, particularly with respect to targeted radionuclide therapy. Similar to NETs, there are numerous studies confirming the powerful prognostic role of FDG PET/CT for thyroid cancer. In a large retrospective series of 400 patients with metastatic thyroid cancer followed for a median of 7.9 years, only age and FDG PET results (SUVmax of the most active lesion and number of FDG-avid lesions) were strong predictors of survival.[2] The American Joint Committee on Cancer stage was not significant in multivariate analysis. Similar findings were reported by Deandreis and colleagues,[31] with FDG uptake as the only significant prognostic factor for survival, without any correlation between histologic subtype, ^{131}I/FDG uptake pattern, or patient outcome. Consequently, the real-time prognostic value of FDG PET/CT should be used at diagnosis of metastatic DTC to guide the aggressiveness of therapy. It has been increasingly recognized that a proportion of patients with indolent metastatic disease can have long-term survival without ongoing treatment after initial surgery and radioiodine therapy,[32] although others warrant aggressive multimodality treatment. Thus, in patients with favorable prognosis as defined by FDG PET/CT, observation, rather than repeated dosing of ^{131}I or tyrosine kinase inhibitor therapy, may be the most appropriate.

Negative Iodine Scan and Increasing Thyroglobulin Levels

In the context of a negative iodine scan and increasing thyroglobulin (Tg) level, FDG PET/CT has high accuracy for detection of residual or recurrent disease. A meta-analysis of 165 patients from 6 studies identified a pooled sensitivity of 93.5% and specificity of 83.9% of PET/CT for detecting disease recurrence, which was superior to conventional techniques.[33] A threshold stimulated Tg level of 10 ng/mL for performing FDG PET/CT is recommended in the American Thyroid Association

DTC management guidelines[34] as a good compromise between sensitivity and specificity. However, a recent series of 102 patients with a positive FDG PET/CT scan result demonstrated that 88% had a Tg greater than 5.5 ng/mL,[35] recognizing that more aggressive dedifferentiated disease may not have a high Tg level. The potential impact of anti-Tg antibodies should also be considered.

The blind administration of ^{131}I in patients with an elevated Tg commits approximately 50% of patients to unnecessary radiation exposure without clinical benefit. Instead, we use a combination of diagnostic iodine (^{123}I SPECT/CT or [124]I PET/CT) and FDG PET/CT imaging to determine suitability for ^{131}I radionuclide therapy, in a manner similar to the theranostic approach for GEP-NETs using PRRT described earlier. Pretherapeutic diagnostic assessment also provides the opportunity for a prospective estimate of dosimetry if suitable for treatment. A pattern of FDG-negative iodine-positive or concordant FDG-positive iodine-positive uptake is typically necessary for therapy (Fig. 6). Any FDG-positive iodine-negative dedifferentiated disease determines the patient's overall prognosis and is not targeted by radionuclide therapy (Fig. 7). Other treatments such as surgery, external beam radiotherapy, and multikinase inhibitor therapy need to be considered to target discordant dedifferentiated FDG-avid disease.

This approach using a pretherapy assessment of combined [124]I and FDG PET/CT scans was described in a series of 19 patients with rising stimulated Tg levels (>9 ng/mL) and no evidence of disease on other imaging modalities.[36] This result lead to disease restaging in 7 of 19 patients and management change in 6 of 19 patients. The primary advantage of this approach was avoidance of unnecessary radiation exposure from blind therapy with [131]I. This approach is being investigated in the multicenter prospective observational THYROPET study using the combination of [124]I and FDG PET/CT in patients with biochemically suspected recurrence of DTC.[37] In patients with confirmed FDG-avid disease, FDG PET/CT also has an important role to play in the evaluation of treatment response.

Is Thyroid-Stimulating Hormone Stimulation Necessary for Fluorodeoxyglucose PET/Computed Tomography in Differentiated Thyroid Cancer?

Although there is a clear benefit in imaging iodine uptake in thyroid cancer under thyroid-stimulating hormone (TSH) stimulation, there is less of a case for the need of TSH stimulation before FDG PET/CT. Although most studies

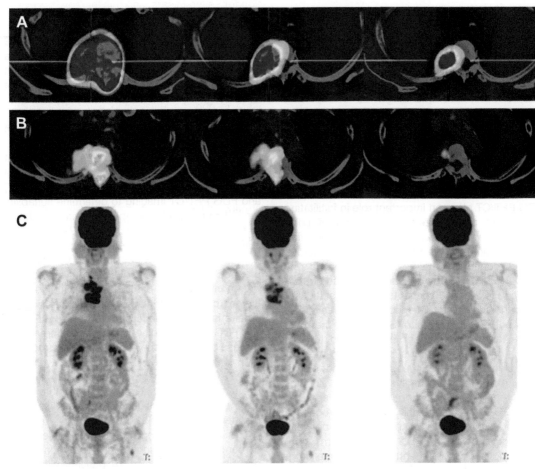

Fig. 6. Concordant iodine-avid/FDG-avid metastatic follicular thyroid carcinoma with excellent metabolic and scintigraphic response to ^{131}I therapy. A 67-year-old man presented with incipient spinal cord compression at T2 from a large upper thoracic mass. He was treated with 7.4 GBq, 5.3 GBq, and 3.0 GBq of I 131 at approximately yearly intervals. Sequential fused axial TSH stimulated ^{123}I SPECT/CT (A) and FDG PET/CT (B) images through the dominant T2 mass and FDG PET maximum intensity projections (C) demonstrate markedly improved ^{123}I appearances and a near-complete metabolic response, highlighting the utility of FDG PET/CT for radionuclide treatment selection and response assessment.

demonstrate an increment in the number of lesions identified, there is low management impact (6%)[38] and the overall clinical significance of these results is unknown. Theoretically, the most poorly differentiated disease will have lost expression of the TSH receptor (and sensitivity to TSH stimulation) in addition to the Na/iodide symporter, rendering TSH stimulation unnecessary. Consequently, these dedifferentiated lesions do not benefit from thyroxine suppression and may warrant a more aggressive treatment approach. In contrast, the small incremental number of hypermetabolic lesions identified after TSH stimulation demonstrates a physiologic response to TSH, representing an intermediate degree of differentiation and more likely to benefit from ongoing thyroxine suppression. These lesions are also identified/treated with iodine imaging/therapy,

and the lack of FDG uptake is unlikely to influence management in this context, which is determined by identification of dedifferentiated non–iodine-avid disease. In any case, most FDG PET/CT studies at our institution are performed concurrently with iodine imaging (and thus TSH stimulation). However, if performed independently, we do not routinely perform TSH stimulation for the reasons outlined earlier.

ROLE OF FLUORODEOXYGLUCOSE PET/CT IN THE MANAGEMENT OF MEDULLARY THYROID CANCER

MTC accounts for approximately 4% of all thyroid cancers, with an overall 10-year survival of between 40% and 80%. Given the side-effect profile of the limited available therapeutic options, it is

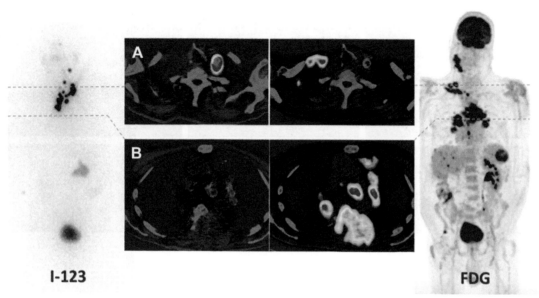

I-123   FDG

Fig. 7. Metastatic papillary thyroid carcinoma with disease heterogeneity demonstrating the flip-flop phenomenon in a pattern such that ^{131}I therapy is unlikely to provide significant clinical benefit. A 71-year-old man with metastatic papillary thyroid cancer being assessed for treatment with ^{131}I therapy versus external beam radiotherapy to large T6 mass. Comparative TSH-stimulated ^{123}I SPECT/CT and FDG PET/CT demonstrate the flip-flop phenomenon; only a small minority of the disease burden is FDG negative iodine positive (including calcified left superior mediastinal lymph nodes, *A*), whereas most disease sites (including large invasive mass at T6 level, *B*) are intensely FDG avid and iodine negative. Consequently, this patient was not suitable for treatment with ^{123}I therapy and received external beam radiotherapy to the T6 lesion.

important to identify those patients at highest risk of disease progression and disease-specific mortality. Calcitonin and carcinoembryonic antigen (CEA) are tumor markers for MTC, and doubling times of these markers are considered the best available indicators to assess progressive disease, MTC recurrence, and cancer mortality.[39] However, the levels can fluctuate and determination of the doubling time requires serial measurement for up to 24 months during which time disease progression may become self-evident. A study of 40 patients by Verbeek and colleagues[40] demonstrated that 77% of FDG-avid patients had a calcitonin/CEA doubling time of less than 24 months identifying patients with poor survival, whereas 88% of FDG-negative patients had a tumor marker doubling time of greater than 24 months. Although ^{18}F-dihydroxyphenylalanine (DOPA) PET/CT was more able to accurately assess the extent of disease, it had less prognostic value. In a small subset of patients in another study with a short calcitonin doubling time of less than 12 months,[41] FDG PET/CT was a better diagnostic test than ^{18}F-DOPA PET/CT, likely representing the extent of dedifferentiated disease and poor prognosis in this group (**Fig. 8**).

The role of FDG PET/CT in radionuclide therapy is less established in the literature for MTC than for GEP-NETs or DTC. Although ^{18}F-DOPA PET/CT demonstrates the best diagnostic utility,[42] its management impact is limited to identifying potentially resectable sites of disease, as it does not have a theranostic pair for radionuclide treatment. Use of SSTR PET/CT can identify a group of patients who potentially benefit from PRRT.[43] In these cases, FDG PET/CT is used in a role similar to that in GEP-NETs and DTC for exclusion of discordant disease and prognostication to guide the intensity of therapy and schedule of follow-up. Other theranostic agents such as gastrin receptor targeting[44] are emerging for this serious condition with limited therapeutic options.

ROLE OF FLUORODEOXYGLUCOSE PET/COMPUTED TOMOGRAPHY IN THE MANAGEMENT OF PHEOCHROMOCYTOMA AND PARAGANGLIOMA

PPGLs are rare catecholamine-producing tumors of the adrenal medulla and extra-adrenal sympathetic chromaffin tissues. A significant proportion of PPGLs has a hereditary basis with specific tumor phenotypes, including catecholamine profile, tumor location, propensity for multiple tumors, and malignant potential; Succinate dehydrogenase subunit B (SDHB) mutations are associated

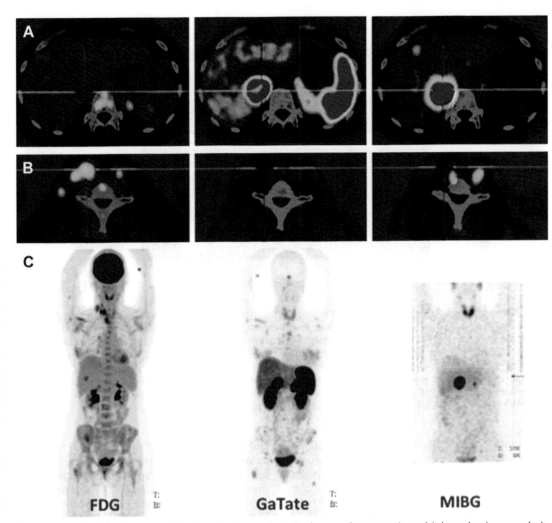

Fig. 8. Molecular imaging accurately characterizes metastatic disease phenotype in multiple endocrine neoplasia, with a poor prognosis predicted by FDG avidity. A 34-year-old woman referred for assessment of radionuclide therapy for metastatic pheochromocytoma with CT scan findings of a 4-cm right adrenal nodule (markedly elevated metanephrines) and multiple osseous/hepatic metastases. Molecular imaging was performed with ^{18}F FDG PET/CT (*column 1*), ^{68}Ga DOTATATE PET/CT (*column 2*), and ^{123}I MIBG SPECT/CT (*column 3*); this demonstrated bilateral DOTATATE- and MIBG-avid adrenal masses, without any FDG uptake, consistent with a cluster 2 genotype pheochromocytoma (*A*). However, there was evidence of a locally invasive mildly FDG-avid right thyroid mass with regional nodal and distant hepatic/osseous metastases sharing the same mildly FDG-avid metabolic signature (*B*). Diagnosis of bilateral pheochromocytoma and metastatic medullary thyroid carcinoma with MEN2A phenotype was established before biopsy. Baseline FDG uptake was highly prognostic with subsequent calcitonin doubling less than 6 months, and the patient died approximately 7 months after diagnosis from metastatic medullary thyroid carcinoma. Maximum intensity projection (MIP) images contrasting the three modalities are shown (*C*).

with a particularly malignant phenotype[45] (**Fig. 9**). As outlined earlier, these hereditary syndromes are divided into the pseudohypoxic cluster 1 (characterized by constitutive activation of HIF and consequent upregulation of glycolysis and FDG avidity, including SDHx and VHL syndrome) and cluster 2, which is associated with defects in genes associated with kinase signaling pathways (including MEN2, NF1, MAX, and TMEM127).

Tumors in the pseudohypoxic cluster invariably have high-intensity metabolic activity enabling a high sensitivity for staging or restaging.[46] The intensity of FDG PET/CT uptake, however, has limited prognostic value, as tumors with an indolent phenotype and low proliferative index still have intense uptake.[47] Moreover, SDHB-associated tumors do carry the worst prognosis, and other factors including temporal change and discordance

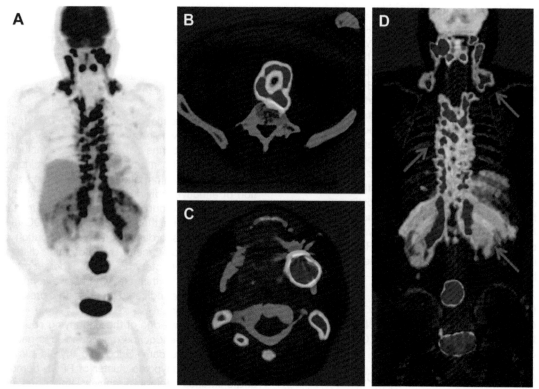

Fig. 9. Molecular imaging phenotype of SDHB-associated metastatic paraganglioma. A 44-year-old man referred for staging of undifferentiated neuroendocrine tumor following biopsy of painful mandible metastasis. FDG PET maximum intensity projection (*A*) and axial PET/CT images demonstrate intensely FDG-avid organ of Zuckerkandl lesion (*B*) and multiple osseous metastases including mandible (*C*). Presence of extensive intensely FDG-avid activated brown fat (*D, blue arrows*) raised the prospect of functioning metastatic paraganglioma, which was subsequently biochemically confirmed. All sites of disease were intensely ^{68}Ga-DOTA-octreotate avid but ^{123}I-MIBG negative (not shown), guiding subsequent treatment with ^{177}Lu-DOTA-octreotate with excellent clinical, biochemical, and scintigraphic response.

with SSTR expression are clues to tumor dedifferentiation.

The presence of intense FDG-avid activated brown fat is well described (but easily overlooked) in patients with catecholamine-producing PPGL (see **Fig 9**)[48]; this may provide an important clue to the diagnosis in the appropriate clinical context such as assessment of adrenal or paravertebral mass or in a patient presenting with an undifferentiated NET. Brown fat may interfere with assessment of distant metastatic disease, which may be overcome by comparison with another molecular imaging modality (eg, ^{68}Ga-DOTA-octreotate) or repeat FDG imaging after administration of combined alpha- and beta-blockade. However, isolated beta-blockade, which is commonly used for brown fat suppression, is contraindicated, as it may precipitate hypertensive crisis due to unopposed α-adrenergic activation.

There is significant variation between reported imaging accuracy for different molecular imaging

tracers for assessment of PPGL. Although some of this variation can be attributed to different imaging modalities (planar vs SPECT vs SPECT/CT vs PET/CT) and physical imaging characteristics of tracers targeting the same metabolic pathway (^{123}I-MIBG vs ^{131}I-MIBG or ^{111}In-octreotide vs ^{68}Ga-DOTA-octreotate), it is likely that selection bias in patient populations (with resultant variable mix of metastatic/localized, hereditary/sporadic, and cluster 1 or 2 tumors) significantly influences the relative accuracy in different studies. The variable imaging phenotypes of the different clinical presentations and suspected underlying genotypes have been categorized in the 2012 European Association of Nuclear Medicine imaging guidelines for PPGL.[49] Our preference based on availability, experience, and theranostic utility with PRRT is to use ^{68}Ga-DOTA-octreotate as an initial diagnostic test.

Targeted radionuclide therapy for metastatic PPGL is well established using ^{131}I-MIBG and an emerging role with PRRT. The principles guiding the use of FDG PET/CT for radionuclide therapy for PPGL are similar to those previously described for NETs. All of our patients with metastatic disease being considered for radionuclide therapy are imaged with ^{123}I (or ^{124}I) MIBG SPECT/CT (or PET/CT), ^{68}Ga-DOTA-octreotate, and FDG PET/CT. The distribution of uptake at identified sites of disease is compared to identify the tracer providing optimal dosimetry and targeting of lesions or evidence of discordant FDG-avid disease. There are well-recognized limitations of ^{123}I-MIBG imaging of metastatic PPGL,[47] and consequently, the SSTR theranostic pair is more frequently used for targeted radionuclide therapy for PPGL in our institution. Sandwich or combined therapy with both MIBG and PRRT has been used in some patients because of metastatic disease heterogeneity.

ROLE OF FLUORODEOXYGLUCOSE PET/ COMPUTED TOMOGRAPHY IN THE MANAGEMENT OF ADRENOCORTICAL CARCINOMA

Adrenocortical carcinoma (ACC) is a rare and aggressive malignancy, variably associated with endocrinopathy (typically rapidly progressive Cushing syndrome with or without virilization in adults), high rates of morbidity/mortality,[50] and limited treatment options. Standard therapy is currently complete surgical resection with adjuvant mitotane or combination chemotherapy for unresectable or metastatic disease with significant toxicity and poor outcomes. A limited number of studies have assessed the utility of FDG PET/CT in ACC and have demonstrated comparably favorable diagnostic value as thoracoabdominopelvic CT (particularly with detection of distant metastatic disease and local recurrence)[51] and substantial change in management in a small number of patients (<10%).[52] Lebouleux and colleagues[51] demonstrated that intensity of FDG uptake (SUV-max >10) and volume of FDG uptake (>150 mL) were significant prognostic factors for survival; however, this was not replicated in a more recent study.[53] The flip-flop phenomenon (between FDG PET/CT and ^{131}I-nor-cholesterol) has also been described in a patient with metastatic ACC.[54]

Targeted radionuclide therapy with the theranostic pair ^{123}I/^{131}I-metomidate has been described in a series of 11 patients, with a favorable median progression-free survival in patients responding to treatment of 14 months and minimal toxicity.[55] FDG PET/CT was used in 7 patients, demonstrating utility in assessing suitability for therapy (excluding sites of dedifferentiated disease) and

response assessment. Further prospective evaluation of this promising targeted radionuclide therapy is warranted with utilization of FDG PET/CT according to the principles outlined earlier.

SUMMARY

The high prognostic value of FDG PET/CT facilitates accurate whole-body disease characterization of endocrine malignancies, including GEP-NETs, DTC, medullary thyroid carcinoma, and PPGL. This information is critical to the selection of effective individualized treatments for this heterogeneous group of diseases, particularly targeted radionuclide therapy, if no sites of FDG-avid disease are discordant from the distribution of theranostic radiotracer. Symptomatic disease (local pain or refractory hormonal hypersecretion) is an exception to this rule, whereby radionuclide therapy may be indicated despite the presence of discordant disease.

A sound knowledge of the underlying cause of FDG uptake in endocrine malignancies is necessary to optimize care. Oncocytic thyroid tumors and the pseudohypoxic cluster of PPGL demonstrate intense metabolic activity that does not necessarily correspond to dedifferentiated disease, and benign causes of FDG uptake must also be considered when assessing suitability for radionuclide therapy. FDG PET/CT also plays an important role in the response assessment of these treatments.

REFERENCES

1. Adams S, Baum R, Rink T, et al. Limited value of fluorine-18 fluorodeoxyglucose positron emission tomography for the imaging of neuroendocrine tumors. Eur J Nucl Med 1998;25:79–83.
2. Robbins RJ, Wan Q, Grewal RK, et al. Real-time prognosis for metastatic thyroid carcinoma based on 2-[18F]fluoro-2-deoxy-D-glucose-positron emission tomography scanning. J Clin Endocrinol Metab 2006;91:498–505.
3. Longo DL. Tumor heterogeneity and personalized medicine. N Engl J Med 2012;366:956–7.
4. Warburg O. On the origin of cancer cells. Science 1956;123:309–14.
5. Feine U, Lietzenmayer R, Hanke JP, et al. 18FDG whole-body PET in differentiated thyroid carcinoma. Flipflop in uptake patterns of 18FDG and I131. Nuklearmedizin 1995;34:127–34.
6. Kelders A, Kennes LN, Krohn T, et al. Relationship between positive thyroglobulin doubling time and 18F-FDG PET/CT positive, 131I-negative lesions. Nucl Med Commun 2014;35:176–81.

7. Taieb D, Sebag F, Barlier A, et al. 18F-FDG avidity of phaeochromocytomas and paragangliomas: a new molecular imaging signature? J Nucl Med 2009;50: 711–7.

8. van Berkel A, Rao JU, Kusters B, et al. Correlation between in vivo 18F-FDG PET and immunohistochemical markers of glucose uptake and metabolism in phaeochromocytoma and paraganglioma. J Nucl Med 2014;55:1253–9.

9. Deandreis D, Al Ghuzlan A, Auperin A, et al. Is 18F-fluorodeoxyglucose-PET/CT useful for the presurgical characterisation of thyroid nodules with indeterminate fine needle aspiration cytology? Thyroid 2012;22:165–72.

10. Zandieh S, Pokieser W, Knoll P, et al. Oncocytic adenomas of thyroid-mimicking benign or metastatic disease on 18F-FDG-PET scan. Acta Radiol 2015; 56:709–13.

11. Gasparre G, Porcelli AM, Bonora E, et al. Disruptive mitochondrial DNA mutations in complex I subunits are markers of oncocytic phenotype in thyroid tumors. Proc Natl Acad Sci U S A 2007; 104:9001–6.

12. Geijer H, Breimer LH. Somatostatin receptor PET/CT in neuroendocrine tumors: update on systematic review and meta-analysis. Eur J Nucl Med Mol Imaging 2013;40:1770–80.

13. Hofman MS, Kong G, Neels OC, et al. High management impact of Ga-68 DOTATATE (GaTate) PET/CT for imaging neuroendocrine and other somatostatin expressing tumors. J Med Imaging Radiat Oncol 2012;56:40–7.

14. Hofman MS, Hicks RJ. Changing paradigms with molecular imaging of neuroendocrine tumors. Discov Med 2012;14:71–81.

15. Kubota K, Okasaki M, Minamimoto R, et al. Lesion-based analysis of (18)F-FDG uptake and (111)In-pentetreotide uptake by neuroendocrine tumors. Ann Nucl Med 2014;28:1004–10.

16. Has Simsek D, Kuyumcu S, Turkmen C, et al. Can complementary 68Ga-DOTATATE and 18F-FDG PET/CT establish the missing link between histopathology and therapeutic approach in gastroenteropancreatic neuroendocrine tumors? J Nucl Med 2014;55:1811–7.

17. Klimstra DS, Modlin IR, Coppola D, et al. The pathologic classification of neuroendocrine tumors: a review of nomenclature, grading, and staging systems. Pancreas 2010;39:707–12.

18. Vander Heiden MG, Cantley LC, Thompson CB. Understanding the Warburg effect: the metabolic requirements of cell proliferation. Science 2009;324: 1029–33.

19. Hofman MS, Hick RJ. Peptide receptor radionuclide therapy for neuroendocrine tumours: standardized and randomized, or personalized? Eur J Nucl Med Mol Imaging 2014;41:211–3.

20. Binderup T, Knigge U, Loft A, et al. 18F-fluorodeoxyglucose positron emission tomography predicts survival of patients with neuroendocrine tumors. Clin Cancer Res 2010;16:978–85.

21. Bahri H, Laurence L, Edeline J, et al. High prognostic value of 18F-FDG PET for metastatic gastroenteropancreatic neuroendocrine tumors: a long-term evaluation. J Nucl Med 2014;55:1786–90.

22. Ezziddin S, Adler L, Sabet A, et al. Prognostic stratification of metastatic gastroenteropancreatic neuroendocrine neoplasms by 18F-FDG PET: feasibility of a metabolic grading system. J Nucl Med 2014;55: 1260–6.

23. Kwekkeboom DJ, de Herder WW, Kam BL, et al. Treatment with the radiolabeled somatostatin analog [177 Lu-DOTA 0,Tyr3]octreotate: toxicity, efficacy, and survival. J Clin Oncol 2008;26:2124–30.

24. Kashyap R, Hofman MS, Michael M, et al. Favourable outcomes of Lu-octreotate peptide receptor chemoradionuclide therapy in patients with FDG-avid neuroendocrine tumors. Eur J Nucl Med Mol Imaging 2015;42:176–85.

25. Claringbold PG, Price RA, Turner JH. Phase I-II study of radiopeptide 177Lu-octreotate in combination with capecitabine and temozolomide in advanced low-grade neuroendocrine tumors. Cancer Biother Radiopharm 2012;27:561–9.

26. Eisenhauer EA, Therasse P, Bogaerts J, et al. New response evaluation criteria in solid tumors: revised RECIST guideline (version 1.1). Eur J Cancer 2009; 45:228–47.

27. Severi S, Nanni O, Bodei L, et al. Role of 18FDG PET/CT in patients treated with 177Lu-DOTATATE for advanced differentiated neuroendocrine tumours. Eur J Nucl Med Mol Imaging 2013;40:881–8.

28. Schlumberger M, Tubania M, Vathaire De, et al. Long-term results of treatment of 283 patients with lung and bone metastases from differentiated thyroid carcinoma. J Clin Endocrinol Metab 1986;63: 960–7.

29. Treglia G, Annunziata S, Muoio B, et al. The role of fluorine-18-fluorodeoxyglucose positron emission tomography in aggressive histological subtypes of thyroid cancer: an overview. Int J Endocrinol 2013; 2013:856189.

30. Pryma DA, Schoder H, Gonen M, et al. Diagnostic accuracy and prognostic value of 18F-FDG PET in Hürthle cell thyroid cancer patients. J Nucl Med 2006;47:1260–6.

31. Deandreis D, Al Ghuzlan A, Leboulleux S, et al. Do histological, immunohistochemical, and metabolic (radioiodine and fluorodeoxyglucose uptakes) patterns of metastatic thyroid cancer correlate with patient outcome? Endocr Relat Cancer 2011;18: 159–69.

32. Kwong N, Marqusee E, Gordon MS, et al. Long-term, treatment-free survival in select patients with

distant metastatic papillary thyroid cancer. Endocr Connect 2014;3:207–14.

33. Dong MJ, Liu ZF, Zhao K, et al. Value of 18FDG-PET/PET-CT in differentiated thyroid carcinoma with radioiodine-negative whole-body scan: a meta-analysis. Nucl Med Commun 2009;30:639–50.

34. Cooper DS, Doherty GM, Haugen BR, et al. Revised American Thyroid Association management guidelines for patients with thyroid nodules and differentiated thyroid cancer. Thyroid 2009;19:1167–214.

35. Giovanella L, Trimboli P, Verburg FA, et al. Thyroglobulin levels and thyroglobulin doubling time independently predict a positive 18F-FDG PET/CT scan in patients with biochemical recurrence of differentiated thyroid carcinoma. Eur J Nucl Med Mol Imaging 2013;40:874–80.

36. Lee J, Nah KY, Kim RM, et al. Effectiveness of [124I]-PET/CT and [18F]-FDG-PET/CT for localizing recurrence in patients with differentiated thyroid carcinoma. J Korean Med Sci 2012;27:1019–26.

37. Kist JW, de Keizer B, Stokkel MP, et al. Recurrent differentiated thyroid cancer: towards personalized treatment based on evaluation of tumor characteristics with PET (THYROPET study): study protocol of a multicenter observational cohort study. BMC Cancer 2014;14:405–13.

38. Leboulleux S, Schroeder PR, Busaidy NL, et al. Assessment of the incremental value of recombinant thyrotropin stimulation before 2-[18F]-fluoro-2-deoxy-D-glucose positron emission tomography/computed tomography imaging to localise residual differentiated thyroid cancer. J Clin Endocrinol Metab 2009;94:1310–6.

39. Meijer JA, le Cessie S, van den Hout WB, et al. Calcitonin and carinoembryonic antigen doubling times as prognostic factors in medullary thyroid carcinoma: a structured meta-analysis. Clin Endocrinol (Oxf) 2010;72:534–42.

40. Verbeek HH, Plukker JT, Koopmans KP, et al. Clinical relevance of 18F-FDG PET and 18F-DOPA PET in recurrent medullary thyroid carcinoma. J Nucl Med 2012;53:1863–71.

41. Koopmans KP, de Groot JW, Plukker JT, et al. 18F-dihydroxyphenylalanine PET in patients with biochemical evidence of medullary thyroid cancer: relation to tumor differentiation. J Nucl Med 2008;49:524–31.

42. Treglia G, Castaldi P, Villani MF, et al. Comparison of 18F-DOPA, 18F-FDG and 68Ga-somatostatin analogue PET/CT in patients with recurrent medullary thyroid carcinoma. Eur J Nucl Med Mol Imaging 2012;39:569–80.

43. Vaisman F, de Castro PH, Lopes FP, et al. Is there a role for peptide receptor radionuclide therapy in medullary thyroid cancer? Clin Nucl Med 2015;40:123–7.

44. Kolenc-Peitl P, Mansi R, Tamma M, et al. Highly improved metabolic stability and pharmacokinetics of indium-111-DOTA-gastrin conjugates for targeting of the gastrin receptor. J Med Chem 2011;54:2602–9.

45. Timmers HJ, Kozupa A, Eisenhofer G, et al. Clinical presentations, biochemical phenotypes, and genotype-phenotype correlations in patients with SDHB-associated pheochromocytomas and paragangliomas. J Clin Endocrinol Metab 2007;92:779–86.

46. Timmers HJ, Chen CC, Carrasquillo JA, et al. Staging and functional characterisation of pheochromocytoma and paraganglioma by 18F-fluorodeoxyglucose (18F-FDG) positron emission tomography. J Natl Cancer Inst 2012;104:700–8.

47. Taieb D, Timmers HJ, Shulkin BL, et al. Renaissance of 18F-FDG positron emission tomography in the imaging of pheochromocytoma/paraganglioma. J Clin Endocrinol Metab 2014;99:2337–9.

48. Yamaga LY, Thom AF, Wagner J, et al. The effect of catecholamines on the glucose uptake in brown adipose tissue demonstrated by (18)F-FDG PET/CT in a patient with adrenal pheochromocytoma. Eur J Nucl Med Mol Imaging 2008;35:446–7.

49. Taieb D, Timmers HJ, Hindie E, et al. EANM 2012 guidelines for radionuclide imaging of phaeochromocytoma and paraganglioma. Eur J Nucl Med Mol Imaging 2012;39:1977–95.

50. Fassnacht M, Johanssen S, Quinkler M, et al. Limited prognostic value of the 2004 International Union against Cancer staging classification for adrenocortical carcinoma: proposal for a revised TNM classification. Cancer 2009;115:243–50.

51. Leboulleux S, Dromain C, Bonniaud G, et al. Diagnostic and prognostic value of 18-fluorodeoxyglucose positron emission tomography in adrenocortical carcinoma: a prospective comparison with computed tomography. J Clin Endocrinol Metab 2006;91:920–5.

52. Takeuchi S, Balachandran A, Habra MA, et al. Impact of 18F-FDG PET/CT on the management of adrenocortical carcinoma: analysis of 106 patients. Eur J Nucl Med Mol Imaging 2014;41:2066–73.

53. Tessonnier L, Ansquer C, Bournaud C, et al. 18F-FDG uptake at initial staging of the adrenocortical cancers: a diagnostic tool but not of prognostic value. World J Surg 2013;37:107–12.

54. Ghander C, Tissier F, Tenenbaum F, et al. A concomitant false-negative 18F-FDG PET imaging in an adrenocortical carcinoma and a high uptake in a corresponding liver metastasis. J Clin Endocrinol Metab 2012;97:1096–7.

55. Hahner S, Kreissl MC, Fassnacht M, et al. [131I]Iodometomidate for targeted radionuclide therapy of advanced adrenocortical carcinoma. J Clin Endocrinol Metab 2012;97:914–22.

Application and Dosimetric Requirements for Gallium-68–labeled Somatostatin Analogues in Targeted Radionuclide Therapy for Gastroenteropancreatic Neuroendocrine Tumors

David Taïeb, MD, PhD[a,b,c,*], Philippe Garrigue, PharmD[d],
Manuel Bardiès, PhD[e], Ahmad Esmaeel Abdullah, MD[a],
Karel Pacak, MD, PhD, DSc[f]

KEYWORDS

- PET • Gallium radioisotopes • Somatostatin • Gastroenteropancreatic • Neuroendocrine

KEY POINTS

- Peptide receptor radionuclide therapy (PRRT) using ^{177}Lu-labeled somatostatin analogues (SSTa) has also shown promise in the treatment of advanced progressive grade 1 and 2 neuroendocrine tumors (NETs).
- PET/computed tomography using gallium-68–labeled SSTa is a prime example of a PET-based theranostic approach that provides prognostic information, selecting good candidates for PRRT, and enabling tumor response assessment for PRRT.
- Theranostics of gastroenteropancreatic NETs based on ^{68}Ga-labeled SSTa PET imaging and targeted therapy applying PRRT with ^{90}Y-labeled and/or ^{177}Lu-labeled SSTa have paved the way for personalized medicine.

CURRENT VIEWS ON THE MOLECULAR ORIGINS OF GASTROENTEROPANCREATIC NEUROENDOCRINE TUMORS

Neuroendocrine tumors (NETs) are neural crest-derived neoplasms with predominant neuroendocrine differentiation and arise in most organs of the body. They account for 0.5% of all malignancies, while the incidence is 2 per 100,000. The most frequent primary sites are the pancreas (pancreatic NET [PanNET]), gastrointestinal tract, and lungs. They share some common

Disclosure: The authors have nothing to disclose.
[a] Department of Nuclear Medicine, La Timone University Hospital, Aix-Marseille University, 264, rue Saint-Pierre, Marseille 13385, France; [b] European Center for Research in Medical Imaging, Aix-Marseille University, Marseille, France; [c] Marseille Cancerology Research Center, Inserm UMR1068, Institut Paoli-Calmettes, Marseille, France; [d] Department of Radiopharmacy, La Timone University Hospital, Aix-Marseille University, Marseille, France; [e] UMR 1037 Inserm/UPS, Cancer Research Center of Toulouse, Toulouse, France; [f] Program in Reproductive and Adult Endocrinology, Eunice Kennedy Shriver National Institute of Child Health & Human Development (NICHD), National Institutes of Health, Bethesda, MD 20892, USA
* Corresponding author. Biophysics and Nuclear Medicine, European Center for Research in Medical Imaging, La Timone University Hospital, Aix-Marseille University, 264, rue Saint-Pierre, Marseille 13385, France.
E-mail address: david.taieb@ap-hm.fr

PET Clin 10 (2015) 477–486
http://dx.doi.org/10.1016/j.cpet.2015.06.001
1556-8598/15/$ – see front matter

biological features, such as overexpression of so-matostatin receptors (SSTRs) in 70% to 100% of cases.

The pathogenesis of most NETs starts with in-herited or somatic driver mutations in the genes that specifically regulate neuroendocrine cell prolif-eration.[1] Exonomic studies of sporadic PanNETs show somatic mutations in the MEN1 (Multiple Endocrine Neoplasia type 1) gene in 44% of these tumors, Daxx (death-domain–associated protein) and ATRX (α-thalassemia/mental retardation syn-drome X-linked) in 43%, and mTOR (mammalian target of rapamycin) pathway genes (PTEN and TSC2) in 14%.[2] Some of the mutations are related to a loss in the integrity of telomere chromatins.[3] Recently, PHLDA3, a repressor of Akt activity, was proposed as a novel tumor suppressor of PanNETs.[4]

The genetic pathogenesis of small intestine NETs (midgut NETs) is less well understood. In contrast with PanNETs, exonomic studies show that somatic mutations are rare in midgut NETs.[5]

CURRENT MANAGEMENT OF METASTATIC GASTROENTEROPANCREATIC NEUROENDOCRINE TUMORS

The management of these tumors relies on several factors, such as the presence of hormones/peptide hypersecretion–related symptoms, tumor stage, and grade. According to the European Neuroendo-crine Tumor Society (ENETS) recommendations, tumors are graded as follows: grade 1 (<2 mito-ses/10 high power field [HPF] on microscopy and <3% Ki67 index); grade 2 (2–20 mitoses/10 HPF or 3%–20% Ki67 index); and grade 3, also called neuroendocrine carcinomas (>20 mitoses/10 HPF or >20% Ki67 index). In the case of disseminated disease, many treatment options are available, with potential associations between systemic and locoregional approaches.

Systemic therapy for patients with progressive metastatic GEP-NETs has historically relied mainly on cytotoxic chemotherapy with some positive re-sponses when using a combination of streptozo-tocin, 5-fluorouracil (5-FU), and doxorubicin (especially in PanNETs). In contrast, these treat-ments had limited efficacy in midgut NETs. There has been breakthrough research in the last few years that has made rapid progress in the targeted therapies of NETs. Because most NETs are hyper-vascular, they can be targeted by antiangiogenic agents. Furthermore, they may also show an acti-vation of the mTOR signaling pathways and be treated with mTOR inhibitors.

In RAD001 in Advanced Neuroendocrine Tu-mors, Third Trial (RADIANT-3), 410 patients with advanced PanNETs and progressive disease were randomly assigned to treatment with oral everolimus 10 mg/d or placebo. Octreotide long-acting release (LAR) was administered at the discretion of the investigators.[6] Everolimus showed improved survival (11.0 months with ever-olimus compared with 4.6 months with the pla-cebo) in the advanced, low-grade (grade 1) or intermediate-grade (grade 2) PanNETs with radio-logical progression.[6] In the RADIANT-2 study, 429 patients with advanced progressive midgut NETs were randomized to receive everolimus 10 mg/d plus octreotide LAR 30 mg/mo or octreotide LAR plus a placebo.[7] In the study, the predefined threshold for statistical significance was not achieved. Therefore, the precise therapeutic activ-ity of everolimus in advanced progressive midgut NETs has not been shown.[7] However, if the tumor was SSTR positive, the CLARINET (Controlled study of Lanreotide Antiproliferative Response in NeuroEndocrine Tumors) trial group has shown that lanreotide is associated with prolonged progression-free survival in patients with metasta-tic midgut and pancreatic NETs of grade 1 or 2.[8] Sunitinib has also been proved to improve progression-free survival and overall survival in pa-tients with advanced PanNETs.[9] In summary, grade 1 and 2 PanNETs and midgut NETs show strikingly different drug response profiles.

SOMATOSTATIN PET/COMPUTED TOMOGRAPHY USING GALLIUM-68–LABELED SOMATOSTATIN ANALOGUES

Well-differentiated NETs often overexpress SSTRs on their cell surfaces that could be targeted for diagnostic and therapeutic purposes by radiolab-eling somatostatin analogues (SSTa). [111]In pen-tetic acid (DTPA) octreotide (Octreoscan, Mallinckrodt Pharmaceuticals, Dublin, Ireland), a synthetic octapeptide labeled with indium-111, was the first radiolabeled SST analogue to be approved for scintigraphy of NETs and has been shown to be well suited for the scintigraphic local-ization of primary and metastatic NETs.[10]

Beyond tumor localization, radionuclide imaging using radiolabeled peptides that target SST may be used to select who is likely to benefit from pep-tide receptor radionuclide therapy (PRRT) and to assess therapeutic responses to PRRT.

Scanning with Octreoscan is usually performed at 4 and 24 hours after tracer injection. Repeat im-aging may be required later. The sensitivity of Oc-treoscan is depends on SST density, tumor grade, and size. In recent years, single-photon emission computed tomography (SPECT)/CT has become more widely available and has the advantage of simultaneous acquisition of both anatomic and functional data, increasing diagnostic confidence in image interpretation and enhancing sensitivity in some cases. Octreoscan scintigraphy is associated with practical constraints such as long imaging times, and gastrointestinal tract artifacts requiring bowel cleansing in some cases. The main disadvantage is the low resolution of the SPECT image, limiting the ability to detect tiny lesions. SPECT also does not provide a quantifiable estimate of the SST expression. Thus, use of PET imaging has been growing rapidly in the localization of paragangliomas, paralleled by great efforts toward the development of new tracers.

The design of the radiotracer (isotope, chelator, peptidic sequence) strongly affects the SST affinity (**Fig. 1**). The generator-produced, positron-emitting gallium-68 (^{68}Ga) is a diagnostic trivalent radiometal with convenient labeling characteristics and is also easily available for the daily routine synthesis of ^{68}Ga-labeled radiopharmaceuticals.

1,4,7,10-Tetraazacyclodecane-1,4,7,10-tetra-acetic acid (DOTA) was identified as a better chelator than DTPA, increasing stability and SST targeting.

Numerous ^{68}Ga-DOTA–conjugated SST analogues have been designed in order to increase affinity of these compounds to SST receptors, but 3 are mostly described: ^{68}Ga-DOTA$_0$-[Tyr^3]octreotide (^{68}Ga-DOTATOC), ^{68}Ga-DOTA$_0$-1-Nal^3-octreotide (^{68}Ga-DOTANOC), and [^{68}Ga-DOTA$_0$-Tyr^3] octreotate (^{68}Ga-DOTATATE). All of these bind to SST2. ^{68}Ga-DOTATATE has been shown to have the highest affinity for STT2 (half maximal inhibitory concentration [IC_{50}] = 0.2 nM vs 2.5 nM for DOTATOC and 1.9 nM for DOTANOC; see **Fig. 1**). DOTANOC also binds specifically to SST3, SST4, and SST5 receptors. DOTATOC binds to SST5, although with lower affinity than DOTANOC.[11–13] In direct comparisons between ^{68}Ga-DOTA-SSTa PET/CT and ^{99m}Tc-HYNIC-Octreotide/^{111}In-pentetreotide SPECT(CT), ^{68}Ga-DOTA-SSTa has performed better than other functional imaging technique, providing a compelling reason for switching from SPECT/CT to PET/CT imaging. PET/CT is also more suitable than SPECT/CT for quantifying the disease at a molecular level.

GALLIUM-68–LABELED SOMATOSTATIN ANALOGUES AS THERANOSTICS FOR GASTROENTEROPANCREATIC NEUROENDOCRINE TUMORS

PRRT has shown promise in the treatment of metastatic grade 1 and 2 NETs.[14,15] ^{90}Y-octreotide and ^{177}Lu-octreotide, have been shown to be efficient and effective therapeutic modalities[16] (**Table** 1). Response rates (mainly partial responses) have been 30% to 60% on average. Disease stabilization is common (20%–50%) but more difficult to interpret.[17–23] Independent predictors of survival in advanced grade 1/2 PanNETs treated by ^{177}Lu-octreotate are the tumor proliferation index, the patient's performance status, tumor burden, and baseline plasma neuron-specific enolase (NSE) level.[23] For advanced NET of the small intestine, tumor functional status and high plasma chromogranin A level seemed to be independent predictors of unfavorable patient outcome.[24]

Randomized clinical trials comparing with other modalities are still lacking.[25]

Trials are ongoing that compare the use of PRRT with ^{177}Lu-octreotate in GEP-NETS with a range of other molecules that were obtained from the database of clinicaltrials.gov.

The CONTROL NETS (Capecitabine On Temozolamide Radionuclide therapy Octreotate Lutetium 177 for Gastroenteropancreatic Neuroendocrine tumors) is an open-label phase 2 study that involves 2 parallel trials, the first comparing PRRT therapy (^{177}Lu-octreotate) plus capecitabine/temozolomide (CAP/TEM) with (1) Lu177-DOTATATE alone in the treatment of low-grade to intermediate-grade midgut NETs; and (2) CAP/TEM alone in the treatment of low-grade to intermediate-grade pancreatic NETs. A further study is assessing treatment with ^{177}Lu-octreotate compared with octreotide LAR in patients with inoperable, progressive, SSTR-positive midgut carcinoid tumors (NETTER-1: First pivotal Phase III study evaluating ^{177}Lu-DOTATATE in midgut neuroendocrine tumors).

The French OCLURANDOM study (Antitumor efficacy of peptide receptor radionuclide therapy with ^{177}Lu-octreotate randomized vs sunitinib in unresectable progressive well-differentiated neuroendocrine pancreatic carcinoma) is a randomized, open-label, multicenter trial that assesses the safety and efficacy of ^{177}Lu-octreotate versus sunitinib in pretreated, progressive, well-differentiated pancreatic NETs and is expected to be finalized in 2023.

Another study is comparing ^{177}Lu-octreotate with interferon alfa-2b in progressive nonpancreatic gastrointestinal NETs that are nonresectable and resistant to therapy with SSTa. The estimated completion date is the end of 2016.

In 2014, the US Food and Drug Administration defined a companion diagnostic device (CDD) as an "*in vitro* [...] or an imaging tool that provides information that is essential for the safe and effective use of a corresponding therapeutic product", publishing an exhaustive list of consequent examples. Most of these were in vitro diagnostic devices like

Octreotide derivative	R₁	R₂	R₃	Radiotracer	sst1	sst2	sst3	sst4	sst5
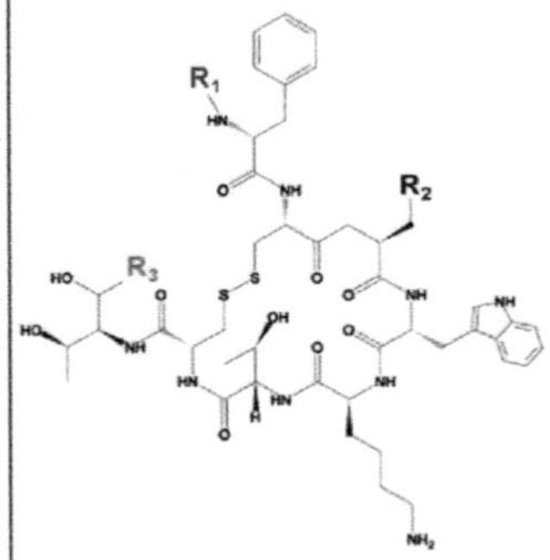	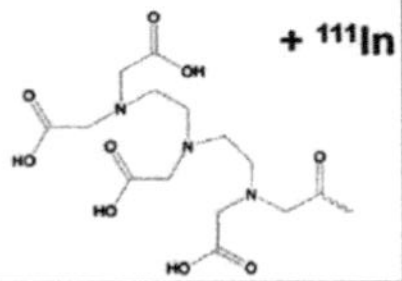 + ^{111}In		—H	^{111}In-pentetreotide	>10,000	22 ±3.6	182 ±13	>1,000	237 ±52
	+ ^{68}Ga or ^{90}Y or ^{177}Lu 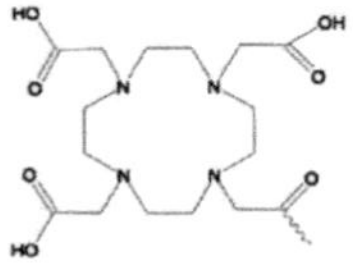	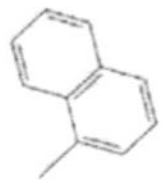	—H	^{68}Ga-DOTANOC	>10,000	1.9 ±0.4	40 ±5.8	260 ±74	7.2 ±1.6
		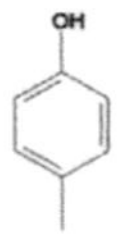	—H	^{68}Ga-DOTATOC	>10,000	2.5 ±0.5	613 ±140	>1,000	73 ±21
			=O	^{68}Ga-DOTATATE	>10,000	0.2 ±0.04	>1,000	300 ±140	377 ±18

Fig. 1. Radiolabeled SSTa with respective affinities for SST subtypes (IC$_{50}$).

Table 1
Pooled number of patients involved in trials regarding different treatment modalities with ^{177}Lu-DOTATATE for NETs (mainly GEP-NETs)

Type of Intervention	Pooled Number of Patients	Number of Studies	CR; N (%)	PR; N (%)	MR; N (%)	SD; N (%)	Favorable Outcome: CR + PR + MR + SD; N (%)	PD; N (%)	Median Progression-free Survival (mo)	Toxicity (%)
^{177}Lu-DOTATATE	988	12	14 (1.4)	310 (31.4)	112 (11.3)	390 (39.5)	826 (83.6)	162 (16.4)	32	Nausea (29–35) Vomiting (10–18) Abdominal discomfort (6–11) Reversible hematotoxicity (5.9–22) Severe nephrotoxicity (1.3)
Retreatment with ^{177}Lu-DOTATATE	88	3	3 (3.4)	10 (11.4)	7 (8)	37 (42)	57 (64.8)	31 (35.2)	18.5	Reversible hematotoxicity (21.2)
Dual treatment: ^{90}Y-DOTATATE plus ^{177}Lu-DOTATATE	88	2	2 (2)	26 (30)	—	45 (51)	73 (83)	15 (17)	18	Reversible hematotoxicity (7–15) G1 renal toxicity (12)

^{177}Lu-DOTATATE combined with chemotherapy	86	2	6 (7)	28 (32)	—	48 (56)	82 (95)	4 (5)	39.5	1. With capecitabine
										  a. Transient hematotoxicity G3/4 (7)
										  b. Mild hand-foot syndrome (9)
										  c. Thrombocytopenia G3 (3)
										2. With temozolomide plus capecitabine
										  a. Nausea (21)
										  b. Transient hematotoxicity G3/4 (16.2)
										  c. Neutropenia G3 (6)
										  d. Thrombocytopenia G2 (24)
										  e. Myelodysplastic syndromes (3)
										3. With 5-FU
										  a. Thrombocytopenia G3/4 (6)
										  b. Hepatotoxicity (11.5)
										  c. Mean yearly reduction in GFR (with renal protection protocol) 2.2 mL/y

Abbreviations: CR, complete remission; GFR, glomerular filtration rate; MR, minor response; PD, progressive disease; PR, partial response; SD, stable disease.

immunohistochemistry and fluorescent in situ hybridization/chromosomal in situ hybridization kits, with the aim of predicting the utility of therapeutic monoclonal antibodies on 1 target (or more) expressed by the tumor. CDDs in imaging, and particularly in PRRT, are emerging.

PET/CT using ^{68}Ga-labeled SST analogues is a prime example of a PET-based theranostic approach. A close correlation was found between maximal standardized uptake value (SUV_{max}) and immunohistochemical scores used for the quantitative assessment of the density of subtypes of SST.[26] The Krenning scale remains the only validated scoring system for selecting good candidates for PRRT.[27] Validation of a new scoring system adapted to ^{68}Ga-DOTA-SSTa PET/CT would be of particular interest.

DOTANOC/DOTATOC/DOTATATE can be radiolabeled with ^{177}Lu for PRRT with a lower energy deposit and a shorter tissue penetration than [90]Y. Note that the same peptide should be used for CDD imaging to avoid potential discordances[28–30] (**Fig. 2**).

PROGNOSTIC VALUE AND TUMOR RESPONSE ASSESSMENT TO PEPTIDE RECEPTOR RADIONUCLIDE THERAPY

PET/CT with ^{68}Ga-DOTA-SSTa might also provide prognostic information. Increased tumor avidity for ^{68}Ga-DOTA-SSTa was associated with prolonged survival.[31] Sequential evaluation of patients with metastatic NET by ^{68}Ga-DOTA-SSTa PET/CT and ^{18}F-fluorodeoxyglucose (FDG) PET/CT, which are often also complementary and indicates the aggressiveness of these tumors, should be recommended at baseline for comprehensive NET grading of patients with these tumors. Patients with high tumor ^{68}Ga-DOTA-SSTa avidity and low ^{18}F-FDG uptake have a better prognosis and are good candidates for PRRT.[27] Decrease in tumor/spleen SUV ratio (and not SUV_{max}) after the first PRRT cycle is associated with a longer progression-free survival,[32] although additional confirmatory studies are needed. However, PRRT in these tumors, in contrast with other tumor types, usually results in smaller tumor size responses

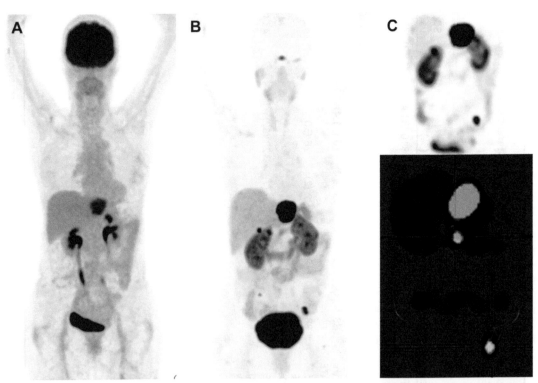

Fig. 2. Molecular imaging of a patient with GEP-NET (PanNET). (*A*) ^{18}F-fluorodeoxyglucose PET/CT (maximal intensity projection [MIP] image). (*B*) ^{68}Ga-DOTATATE PET/CT (MIP image). (*C*) Post–[177]Lu-DOTATATE SPECT/CT imaging: (*top*) MIP, (*middle and bottom*) axial SPECT/CT images centered on the lesions). (*Courtesy of* Christophe Deroose, PhD, Nuclear Medicine, University Hospitals Leuven and Department of Imaging & Pathology, KU Leuven, Belgium.)

compared with functional status responses (eg, done by monitoring secretory status of these tumors), which are often substantial. Thus, Response Evaluation Criteria in Solid Tumors (RECIST) and World Health Organization criteria for classifying tumor response are less adapted to the evaluation of targeted therapies and PRRT because only a small percentage of patients show a significant decline in tumor size despite their clinical and biochemical improvements. Furthermore, it is widely recognized that molecular/functional responses precede morphologic responses and therefore enable an earlier evaluation of overall therapy response.

INTERNAL DOSIMETRY

Internal dosimetry enables a personalized approach to patient treatment. The idea of a common dosimetry protocol applicable to all targeted radionuclide therapy (TRT) procedures is a widespread misconception, possibly derived from the wish to standardize therapeutic applications in nuclear medicine.

TRT dosimetry must be implemented in order to answer a clinical question. Dosimetry implementations, as seen in the literature, are diverse and depend on the clinical context (the aim of the therapy) and the radiopharmaceutical and its mode of administration. In addition, the isotope attached to the biological vector affects the methodology that can be implemented. Safety-related dosimetry focuses on the organs at risk (OARs), whereas efficacy-related dosimetry focuses on tumors.[33]

This is consistent with legal requirements, derived from European Atomic Energy Community (EURATOM) Directive 97/43 and the more recent Directive 2013/59 that states: "For all medical exposure of patients for radiotherapeutic purposes, exposures of target volumes shall be individually planned and their delivery appropriately verified taking into account that doses to non-target volumes and tissues shall be as low as reasonably achievable and consistent with the intended radiotherapeutic purpose of the exposure." In that respect, dosimetry that works should establish the relationship between injected activity and observed biological or clinical effect: "The objective of dosimetry in targeted radionuclide therapy is to provide information that will help improve patient care. With this objective, estimated absorbed dose is useful to the extent that it relates to response."[34] In that sense, dosimetry is the missing link that allows treatment personalization.

The current administration scheme of ^{177}Lu-labeled peptides is based on repeated administrations of fixed activities, most often 4 to 6 cycles of 7.4 GBq of radiopharmaceutical.

- The front-line OAR is the kidney, because toxicity has been observed in that kind of treatment (initially with ^{90}Y-labeled peptides), which explains why the renal function is followed during the course of the treatment. Suspicion of kidney toxicity may lead to a decrease injected activities or may even stop the treatment.
- The second OAR is bone marrow.
- Tumor dosimetry has been reported, even though to date more as a way to document the therapy than as a means to define the posology. However, a significant correlation between absorbed dose and tumor reduction was reported.[35]

Dosimetry that works in PRRT should be designed to assess kidneys, bone marrow, and tumor-absorbed doses, with the aim of establishing the relationship between absorbed dose and observed effect.

Regarding clinical dosimetry, the well-known ^{90}Y-DOTATOC trial yielded important conclusions[36]:

- Activity quantification (and cumulated activity determination) is of paramount importance. [86]Y-DOTATOC was used to assess pharmacokinetics,[37] an important task because [86]Y is a so-called dirty isotope with low positron abundance, and emits a high proportion of single gammas in the range of the coincidence window.[38]
- The model used for absorbed dose calculation also has a major impact: By moving from a standard kidney model for all patients to a better accounting of patient-specific kidney volume, the correlation between absorbed dose and kidney toxicity significantly improved.
- Accounting for radiobiological parameters (computation of the biologically equivalent dose [BED]) allowed further improvement of the correlation. It is remarkable that this was accomplished by deriving BED values from parameters issued from external beam radiotherapy, thereby showing that a robust phenomenon supports the absorbed dose-effect correlation.[39]
- In a retrospective study, Walrand and colleagues also showed a good correlation between red marrow absorbed dose and platelet count reduction at the nadir.[37]

For ^{177}Lu-labeled PRRT, kidney toxicity is less frequent,[20] which can be explained partly by the different range of radiation emitted by ^{177}Lu compared with [90]Y.[40] This difference makes the determination of the absorbed dose (or surrogate)–effect relationship more difficult to characterize.

Dosimetry with ^{177}Lu-labeled peptides, when performed, is usually meant to ensure that the absorbed dose (or surrogate) delivered to kidney does not exceed a certain threshold (safety). Nephrotoxicity is increased in patients with baseline impaired renal function and is more frequently observed in those who develop hematotoxicity during PRRT. Nephroprotection by using positively charged molecules such as L-lysine and/or L-arginine (which competitively inhibit the proximal tubular reabsorption of the radiopeptide) is recommended.

There is usually no pretherapeutic dosimetry: absorbed dose is assessed for every therapy cycle, in order to ensure that the next cycle can be safely administered. This conservative approach relies on the hypothesis that intrapatient pharmacokinetics variability is less than interpatient variability.

On principle, that scheme could be used to modulate injected activity; as is done, for example, in metaiodobenzylguanidine (^{131}I-mIBG) neuroblastoma molecular radiotherapy, in which the absorbed dose assessed for the first, fixed injection (444 MBq/kg) is used to derive the activity to administer for the second injection, under the constraint of limiting the whole-body absorbed dose to less than 4 Gy.[41]

However, ^{177}Lu-labeled PRRT, as currently delivered, is not very toxic; the maximum tolerated absorbed dose has probably not been reached, and therefore it is difficult to provide evidence for absorbed dose-toxicity correlations. A potential reason for the apparent absence of correlation could be that there are methodological flaws in the dosimetric protocol implemented, but a simpler reason could be that the lack of effect limits the possibility of evaluating the dose-response relationship.

The dosimetric protocols implemented have very high heterogeneity, and the comparison and appraisal of uncertainties is difficult.[42]

Most protocols implement two-dimensional whole-body dosimetry at different times after injection (3–7 time points), even though this approach is known to be limited, essentially because of the overlap of source contribution in anterior-posterior projections and the difficulty of correcting for background. Time sampling is also variable, and this is known to markedly affect the determination of cumulated activities.[43] Even for three-dimensional approaches, protocols could not be compared.

A discussion of the current means to derive dosimetry for PRRT is given in an article by Cremonesi and colleagues,[42] who presented the various possibilities offered for pretherapeutic and posttherapeutic dosimetry (see Fig. 2). The possibility of using ^{68}Ga as a surrogate isotope for quantitative imaging PET studies is mentioned. However, because of the very short physical half-life of ^{68}Ga (68 minutes) compared with ^{90}Y and ^{177}Lu, data collection can only be performed for up to a few hours after the injection (see Table 2). In principle, this should rule out ^{68}Ga for dosimetric studies. However, some recent studies highlighted the potential of ^{68}Ga for assessing the response to PRRT,[32,44] which means that the effect of the absorbed dose-effect relationship can be identified. It is therefore tempting to see how ^{68}Ga could be used in a dosimetric context. Velikyan[45] proposed an elegant concept for combining the good activity quantification obtained from ^{68}Ga PET imaging with late data acquisition from ^{177}Lu blood sampling or quantitative SPECT imaging. This approach deserves to be studied. Beyond internal dosimetry, there are also unidentified individual susceptibilities to radiation-associated disease.[46]

SUMMARY

Theranostics of GEP-NETs based on ^{68}Ga-labeled SSTa PET imaging and targeted therapy applying PRRT with ^{90}Y-labeled and/or ^{177}Lu-labeled SSTa has paved the way for personalized medicine (Fig. 3). Future directions include the clinical use of somatostatin antagonists as targeting peptides for imaging and therapy[47] and the development of novel receptor-targeting radiopharmaceuticals that hold promise for theranostics of NETs.

Table 2
Physical characteristics of ^{68}Ga, ^{90}Y, and ^{177}Lu maximum energy of the emitted β particle

	Half-life (h)	Eβ$_{max}$ (Mev)	Maximum Tissue Penetration (mm)
^{68}Ga	1.08	1.9	10
^{90}Y	64.1	2.3	12
^{177}Lu	160.4	0.5	<2

Abbreviation: Eβ$_{max}$, maximum energy of the emitted beta particle.

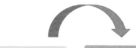

Tissue sampling   Tumor characterization   Management strategy

Tissue analysis   Tumor grading   Determination of prognosis

SST subtypes and   Selection of appropriate peptide
other peptide receptors   for PET imaging
expression profiling

Therapy guidance
Molecular/metabolite/genetic profiling   (PRRT vs other approaches)

Fig. 3. Personalized approach to patients with GEP-NET: from tissue analysis to therapy. (*Adapted from* Baum RP, Kulkarni HR, Carreras C. Peptides and receptors in image-guided therapy: theranostics for neuroendocrine neoplasms. Semin Nucl Med 2012;42(3):190–207; with permission.)

REFERENCES

1. Lewis MA, Yao JC. Molecular pathology and genetics of gastrointestinal neuroendocrine tumours. Curr Opin Endocrinol Diabetes Obes 2014;21(1): 22–7.
2. Jiao Y, Shi C, Edil BH, et al. DAXX/ATRX, MEN1, and mTOR pathway genes are frequently altered in pancreatic neuroendocrine tumors. Science 2011; 331(6021):1199–203.
3. Marinoni I, Kurrer AS, Vassella E, et al. Loss of DAXX and ATRX are associated with chromosome instability and reduced survival of patients with pancreatic neuroendocrine tumors. Gastroenterology 2014;146(2):453–60.e5.
4. Ohki R, Saito K, Chen Y, et al. PHLDA3 is a novel tumor suppressor of pancreatic neuroendocrine tumors. Proc Natl Acad Sci U S A 2014;111(23): E2404–13.
5. Banck MS, Kanwar R, Kulkarni AA, et al. The genomic landscape of small intestine neuroendocrine tumors. J Clin Invest 2013;123(6):2502–8.
6. Yao JC, Shah MH, Ito T, et al. Everolimus for advanced pancreatic neuroendocrine tumors. N Engl J Med 2011;364(6):514–23.
7. Pavel ME, Hainsworth JD, Baudin E, et al. Everolimus plus octreotide long-acting repeatable for the treatment of advanced neuroendocrine tumours associated with carcinoid syndrome (RADIANT-2): a randomised, placebo-controlled, phase 3 study. Lancet 2011;378(9808):2005–12.
8. Caplin ME, Pavel M, Cwikla JB, et al. Lanreotide in metastatic enteropancreatic neuroendocrine tumors. N Engl J Med 2014;371(3):224–33.
9. Raymond E, Dahan L, Raoul JL, et al. Sunitinib malate for the treatment of pancreatic neuroendocrine tumors. N Engl J Med 2011;364(6):501–13.
10. Baum RP, Kulkarni HR, Carreras C. Peptides and receptors in image-guided therapy: theranostics for neuroendocrine neoplasms. Semin Nucl Med 2012; 42(3):190–207.
11. Wild D, Macke HR, Waser B, et al. 68Ga-DOTANOC: a first compound for PET imaging with high affinity for somatostatin receptor subtypes 2 and 5. Eur J Nucl Med Mol Imaging 2005;32(6):724.
12. Wild D, Schmitt JS, Ginj M, et al. DOTA-NOC, a high-affinity ligand of somatostatin receptor subtypes 2, 3 and 5 for labelling with various radiometals. Eur J Nucl Med Mol Imaging 2003;30(10):1338–47.
13. Reubi JC, Schar JC, Waser B, et al. Affinity profiles for human somatostatin receptor subtypes SST1-SST5 of somatostatin radiotracers selected for scintigraphic and radiotherapeutic use. Eur J Nucl Med 2000;27(3):273–82.
14. Ezziddin S, Opitz M, Attassi M, et al. Impact of the Ki-67 proliferation index on response to peptide receptor radionuclide therapy. Eur J Nucl Med Mol Imaging 2011;38(3):459–66.
15. Ezziddin S, Attassi M, Yong-Hing CJ, et al. Predictors of long-term outcome in patients with well-differentiated gastroenteropancreatic neuroendocrine tumors after peptide receptor radionuclide therapy with 177Lu-octreotate. J Nucl Med 2014; 55(2):183–90.
16. Bodei L, Cremonesi M, Kidd M, et al. Peptide receptor radionuclide therapy for advanced neuroendocrine tumors. Thorac Surg Clin 2014;24(3):333–49.
17. Waldherr C, Pless M, Maecke HR, et al. Tumor response and clinical benefit in neuroendocrine tumors after 7.4 GBq (90)Y-DOTATOC. J Nucl Med 2002;43(5):610–6.
18. Kwekkeboom DJ, de Herder WW, Kam BL, et al. Treatment with the radiolabeled somatostatin analog [177 Lu-DOTA 0,Tyr3]octreotate: toxicity, efficacy, and survival. J Clin Oncol 2008;26(13):2124–30.
19. Imhof A, Brunner P, Marincek N, et al. Response, survival, and long-term toxicity after therapy with the radiolabeled somatostatin analogue [90Y-DOTA]-TOC in metastasized neuroendocrine cancers. J Clin Oncol 2011;29(17):2416–23.
20. Bodei L, Cremonesi M, Grana CM, et al. Peptide receptor radionuclide therapy with (1)(7)(7)Lu-DOTA-TATE: the IEO phase I-II study. Eur J Nucl Med Mol Imaging 2011;38(12):2125–35.
21. Danthala M, Kallur KG, Prashant GR, et al. (177)Lu-DOTATATE therapy in patients with neuroendocrine

tumours: 5 years' experience from a tertiary cancer care centre in India. Eur J Nucl Med Mol Imaging 2014;41(7):1319–26.

22. Paganelli G, Sansovini M, Ambrosetti A, et al. 177 Lu-Dota-octreotate radionuclide therapy of advanced gastrointestinal neuroendocrine tumors: results from a phase II study. Eur J Nucl Med Mol Imaging 2014;41(10):1845–51.

23. Ezziddin S, Khalaf F, Vanezi M, et al. Outcome of peptide receptor radionuclide therapy with 177Lu-octreotate in advanced grade 1/2 pancreatic neuroendocrine tumours. Eur J Nucl Med Mol Imaging 2014;41(5):925–33.

24. Sabet A, Dautzenberg K, Haslerud T, et al. Specific efficacy of peptide receptor radionuclide therapy with Lu-octreotate in advanced neuroendocrine tumours of the small intestine. Eur J Nucl Med Mol Imaging 2015;42(8):1238–46.

25. van der Zwan WA, Bodei L, Mueller-Brand J, et al. GEP-NETS update: radionuclide therapy in neuroendocrine tumors. Eur J Endocrinol 2015;172:R1–8.

26. Kaemmerer D, Peter L, Lupp A, et al. Molecular imaging with (6)(8)Ga-SSTR PET/CT and correlation to immunohistochemistry of somatostatin receptors in neuroendocrine tumours. Eur J Nucl Med Mol Imaging 2011;38(9):1659–68.

27. Krenning EP, Kwekkeboom DJ, Bakker WH, et al. Somatostatin receptor scintigraphy with [111In-DTPA-D-Phe1]- and [123I-Tyr3]-octreotide: the Rotterdam experience with more than 1000 patients. Eur J Nucl Med 1993;20(8):716–31.

28. Wild D, Bomanji JB, Benkert P, et al. Comparison of 68Ga-DOTANOC and 68Ga-DOTATATE PET/CT within patients with gastroenteropancreatic neuroendocrine tumors. J Nucl Med 2013;54(3):364–72.

29. Basu S, Abhyankar A, Kand P, et al. 'Reverse discordance' between 68Ga-DOTA-NOC PET/CT and 177Lu-DOTA-TATE posttherapy scan: the plausible explanations and its implications for high-dose therapy with radiolabeled somatostatin receptor analogs. Nucl Med Commun 2011;32(7):654–8.

30. Damle NA, Bal C, Gupta S, et al. Discordance in 68Ga-DOTANOC and 177Lu-DOTATATE uptake in diagnostic and post-therapy scans in patients with medullary thyroid cancer-likely reasons. J Cancer Res Ther 2013;9(4):754–5.

31. Campana D, Ambrosini V, Pezzilli R, et al. Standardized uptake values of (68)Ga-DOTANOC PET: a promising prognostic tool in neuroendocrine tumors. J Nucl Med 2010;51(3):353–9.

32. Haug AR, Auernhammer CJ, Wangler B, et al. 68Ga-DOTATATE PET/CT for the early prediction of response to somatostatin receptor-mediated radionuclide therapy in patients with well-differentiated neuroendocrine tumors. J Nucl Med 2010;51(9):1349–56.

33. Strigari L, Konijnenberg M, Chiesa C, et al. The evidence base for the use of internal dosimetry in the clinical practice of molecular radiotherapy. Eur J Nucl Med Mol Imaging 2014;41(10):1976–88.

34. Sgouros G. Toward patient-friendly cell-level dosimetry. J Nucl Med 2007;48(4):496–7.

35. Ilan E, Sandstrom M, Wassberg C, et al. Dose response of pancreatic neuroendocrine tumors treated with peptide receptor radionuclide therapy using 177Lu-DOTATATE. J Nucl Med 2015;56(2):177–82.

36. Barone R, Borson-Chazot F, Valkema R, et al. Patient-specific dosimetry in predicting renal toxicity with (90)Y-DOTATOC: relevance of kidney volume and dose rate in finding a dose-effect relationship. J Nucl Med 2005;46(Suppl 1):99S–106S.

37. Walrand S, Jamar F, Mathieu I, et al. Quantitation in PET using isotopes emitting prompt single gammas: application to yttrium-86. Eur J Nucl Med Mol Imaging 2003;30(3):354–61.

38. Walrand S, Flux GD, Konijnenberg MW, et al. Dosimetry of yttrium-labelled radiopharmaceuticals for internal therapy: 86Y or 90Y imaging? Eur J Nucl Med Mol Imaging 2011;38(Suppl 1):S57–68.

39. Wessels BW, Konijnenberg MW, Dale RG, et al. MIRD pamphlet no. 20: the effect of model assumptions on kidney dosimetry and response–implications for radionuclide therapy. J Nucl Med 2008;49(11):1884–99.

40. Konijnenberg M, Melis M, Valkema R, et al. Radiation dose distribution in human kidneys by octreotides in peptide receptor radionuclide therapy. J Nucl Med 2007;48(1):134–42.

41. Flux GD, Chittenden SJ, Saran F, et al. Clinical applications of dosimetry for mIBG therapy. Q J Nucl Med Mol Imaging 2011;55(2):116–25.

42. Cremonesi M, Ferrari M, Di Dia A, et al. Recent issues on dosimetry and radiobiology for peptide receptor radionuclide therapy. Q J Nucl Med Mol Imaging 2011;55(2):155–67.

43. Guerriero F, Ferrari ME, Botta F, et al. Kidney dosimetry in (1)(7)(7)Lu and (9)(0)Y peptide receptor radionuclide therapy: influence of image timing, time-activity integration method, and risk factors. Biomed Res Int 2013;2013:935351.

44. Kratochwil C, Stefanova M, Mavriopoulou E, et al. SUV of [(68)Ga]DOTATOC-PET/CT predicts response probability of PRRT in neuroendocrine tumors. Mol Imaging Biol 2015;17(3):313–8.

45. Velikyan I. Prospective of (6)(8)Ga-radiopharmaceutical development. Theranostics 2013;4(1):47–80.

46. Bodei L, Kidd M, Paganelli G, et al. Long-term tolerability of PRRT in 807 patients with neuroendocrine tumours: the value and limitations of clinical factors. Eur J Nucl Med Mol Imaging 2015;42(1):5–19.

47. Wild D, Fani M, Fischer R, et al. Comparison of somatostatin receptor agonist and antagonist for peptide receptor radionuclide therapy: a pilot study. J Nucl Med 2014;55(8):1248–52.

PET/Computed Tomography in the Individualization of Treatment of Prostate Cancer

Francesco Ceci, MD[a],*, Paolo Castellucci, MD[a],
Tiziano Graziani, MD[a], Riccardo Schiavina, MD[b],
Stefano Fanti, MD[a]

KEYWORDS

- Choline PET/CT • Salvage radiotherapy • Salvage lymph-node dissection • PET-guided therapies
- Biochemical relapse

KEY POINTS

- Choline PET/computed tomography (CT) may in patients with relapsed prostate cancer (PCa) show the site of tumor recurrence in a single-step examination, earlier than other conventional imaging techniques.
- Choline PET/CT is used in recurrent PCa to guide personalized therapies in patients with oligometastatic disease.
- The addition of choline PET/CT in the diagnostic flowchart of patients with PCa may affect significantly treatment strategies and patient management.

INTRODUCTION

PCa is the most common malignancy in men in Western Europe and the United States. The incidence has increased in the last few years, and currently PCa is the second most common cause of cancer death in men older than 50 years. Within the European Union, the incidence rate is 78.9 per 100,000 per year and the mortality rate is 30.6 per 100,000 per year. This tumor shows variable biological behavior, from a clinically silent, indolent intraprostatic tumor to an aggressive malignancy.[1] Serum levels of prostate-specific antigen (PSA), digital rectal examination, and transrectal ultrasonography (TRUS)-guided biopsies are usually performed to diagnose and locally stage the disease.[2] Primary treatment depends on age, local and distant staging, surgical risk, and performance status. The most common approaches are radical prostatectomy (RP), external beam radiation therapy (EBRT), brachytherapy (alone or in combination with EBRT), and androgen deprivation therapy (ADT) with adjuvant intent.[2] Several conventional imaging (CI) procedures are available to study patients with PCa: TRUS with or without biopsy, MR imaging, CT, and bone scintigraphy. However, CI proved to have several limitations. In the first diagnosis of local disease, when PCa is suspected, TRUS-guided biopsy can result in negative or inconclusive findings.[3–5] MR imaging with endorectal coil and spectroscopy gave better results than TRUS in the localization of primary cancer.[6–8] Otherwise, the main limitation of MR imaging is related to the low accuracy of MR imaging

The authors have nothing to disclose.

[a] Service of Nuclear Medicine, S.Orsola-Malpighi Hospital, University of Bologna, Via Massarenti 9, 40138 Bologna, Italy; [b] Department of Urology, S.Orsola-Malpighi Hospital, University of Bologna, Via Massarenti 9, 40138 Bologna, Italy

* Corresponding author. Service of Nuclear Medicine, Policlinico S.Orsola-Malpighi, PAD.30, Via Massarenti 9, 40138 Bologna, Italy.

E-mail address: francesco.ceci83@gmail.com

PET Clin 10 (2015) 487–494

http://dx.doi.org/10.1016/j.cpet.2015.05.004

if performed early after TRUS biopsy, which still remains the first diagnostic option.[9,10] During presurgical staging, CI provides information about the local extension of the disease and anatomic information, with MR imaging being considered the gold standard.[11] However, the accuracy of CI is low regarding evaluation of pelvic lymph node (LN) metastasis and distant localizations. LN involvement and distant metastasis are generally presumed according to nomograms.[12] Increasing PSA levels after primary therapy (PSA>0.2 ng/mL after RP or PSA>2 ng/mL more than the nadir after EBRT) are defined as biochemical relapse (BR).[13] BR occurs in 20% to 30% of patients after RP[13,14] and up to 60% after EBRT,[15] and CI modalities did not show optimal performance in the detection of the real site of relapse.[15,16] Consequently, diagnostic workup is recommended by the European Association of Urology only if PSA reaches very high levels (PSA>20 ng/mL).[17]

Functional imaging, in particular PET, demonstrated to be a useful imaging tool, showing molecular function and metabolic activity information that are not available with other modalities.[18] Many tracers labeled with beta-emitter isotopes have been evaluated in PET imaging to choose the most appropriate tracer to investigate patients with PCa.[19] Valid results were obtained in the last years with choline, labeled with C 11 or F 18,[19] a substrate for the synthesis of phosphatedylcholine[20] and with an upregulated expression in PCa cells.[21]

In the initial diagnostic workup before histologic confirmation, choline PET/CT demonstrated limited usefulness, and it is not recommended as a first-line screening method in men at high risk of PCa. Only in patients with high probability of PCa who underwent at least 2 inconclusive prostate biopsies, choline PET/CT could guide TRUS biopsy to the site of higher choline uptake.[22]

During presurgical procedures in patients with high risk of LN involvement already listed for RP, imaging is performed with the intent of better evaluating the real extension of the disease. Considering the suboptimal performance of CT and pelvic MR imaging in the assessment of metastatic LNs and extrapelvic lesions (either visceral or skeletal),[23] choline PET/CT has been proposed.[24] It provided better performance for LN assessment than CI but is still suboptimal to be considered as routine imaging procedure before RP.[24] At present, choline PET/CT cannot be recommended to stage all patients with PCa. Only patients with high risk of distant metastasis that could be excluded from RP considering the presence of LNs outside the pelvis or bone metastasis should be referred to choline PET/CT.[24]

The leading role of PET imaging in PCa is represented by the detection of the site of relapse in patients presenting BR. In this group of patients, it is crucial to differentiate between local and distant relapse to choose the proper treatment strategy.[25] In case of suspicion of prostate bed relapse, patients are addressed to salvage RT (S-RT) with or without nodal irradiation, whereas patients with suspicious systemic metastasis are usually addressed to ADT or other systemic treatment. Choline PET/CT may show the site of tumor recurrence in a single-step examination, earlier than CI techniques,[17] and its detection rate (DR) is related to PSA and PSA kinetics.[26,27] A diagnostic test capable of differentiating potentially curable local recurrence and metastatic disease including distant involvement implying palliative approaches may be able to play an important role in those cases in whom targeted therapies could be performed according to PET results and in patient management.[28]

This review analyzes the value of PET imaging in the evaluation of treatment of patients with PCa. In particular, the different treatment strategies that could be performed are evaluated, according to choline PET results.

CHOLINE PET/COMPUTED TOMOGRAPHY TO GUIDE SALVAGE RADIOTHERAPY

External-beam radiotherapy is considered one of the most diffused treatment approaches as primary therapy together with RP with or without pelvic lymph-node dissection (PLND).[29] Moreover, RT proved to have a valuable role in the treatment of patients with recurrent disease suspected for local relapse.[30,31] For the best chance of success, S-RT on prostate bed must be administered when the cancer burden is low, that is, when PSA first reaches detectable levels.[30,31] Stephenson and colleagues[30] reported a disease-free survival (DFS) at 6 years after S-RT of 40% for patients showing PSA level less than 0.5 ng/mL before the treatment and of 18% for those showing PSA level greater than 1.5 ng/mL. However, most patients treated with S-RT showed BR after salvage treatments.[30,31] For this reason, also at the early phase of BR, all efforts should be made to exclude the presence of distant metastasis, outside of those included in the field of treatment. Castellucci and colleagues[27] investigated with ^{11}C-choline PET/CT a large cohort of patients with recurrent PCa already listed for S-RT in the prostatic bed in an early phase of BR. The study enrolled 605 patients, with PSA levels greater than 0.2 ng/mL and less than 2 ng/mL. The overall PET DR was 28.7% with an incidence of intrapelvic findings of 13.7%

and extrapelvic findings of 14.7%. However, the DR of PET increased dramatically in patients with a PSA doubling-time lower than 6 months (47%) or in patients with ongoing ADT (46%). The investigators reported a statistical association between PET results and PSA level, PSA kinetics, and ongoing ADT at multivariate analysis. They concluded that ^{11}C-choline PET/CT may be suggested before S-RT particularly in patients showing fast PSA kinetics or increasing levels of PSA despite ongoing ADT, considering the higher probability to detect positive findings outside the pelvis. These patients could be excluded from S-RT because of the presence of distant metastases, avoiding futile aggressive treatment and preventing radiation-induced morbidity. Moreover, the detection of positive locoregional LNs on PET/CT could have an impact on patient management performing S-RT in an extended planning target volumes (PTV). The study emphasizes the importance of PET imaging to guide therapies not only on the local recurrence but also in case of LN relapse.

Choline PET/CT could be used for patient risk stratification according to the clinical and imaging features, selecting those patients who are most likely to respond and benefit from aggressive treatments such as S-RT or salvage PLND (S-PLND). Different studies designed to investigate the importance of PET imaging to guide S-RT have been published. Souvatzoglou and colleagues[32] investigated a cohort of 37 patients treated with RP and referred to S-RT to the prostatic fossa because of BR. One-third of the patients had a positive finding at ^{11}C-choline PET/CT, and 13% (5 patients) of the enrolled population showed positive PET findings outside of the prostatic fossa (iliac LNs). S-RT was adjusted according to PET results, implicating an extension of the PTV, including PET-positive LNs. At the end of the follow-up, 56% of patients had a PSA level of 0.2 ng/mL or less, and in the 5 patients in whom the PTV had been enlarged according to PET results, the biochemical relapse-free survival (BFS) rate was 80%. Würschmidt and colleagues[33] reported their results on a population of 19 patients with recurrent PCa treated with intensity-modulated RT for BR after RP. They delivered a standard dose on the prostatic bed with a boost (65 Gy) on ^{18}F-choline PET/CT–positive LNs. After 28 months of follow-up, they reported an overall survival of 94%, a BFS of 49%, and a distant DFS of 75%. They concluded that ^{18}F-choline PET/CT could be helpful in dose escalation in PCa. In their experience, ^{18}F-choline PET/CT allowed a boost dose to metastatic LN regions if image-guided radiotherapy is used. Another promising study has been published by Picchio

and colleagues.[34] They reported similar results using ^{11}C-choline PET/CT for planning and monitoring helical tomotherapy with simultaneous integrated boost in patients presenting only LN relapse at PET imaging. The investigators enrolled 83 patients with recurrent PCa, who underwent irradiation on pelvic or abdominal LNs with a boost (65 Gy) on ^{11}C-choline PET/CT–positive LNs. The main limitation of this study is the short follow-up used to monitor PSA response (mean, 83 days; range, 16–365 days). However, the investigators observed an early biochemical partial response in 70% of cases, and treatment was well tolerated, with grade 3 acute toxicity in the genitourinary tract observed only in 2.4% of the population. D'Angelillo and colleagues[35] investigated a cohort of 60 patients with BR after RP, treated according to ^{18}F-choline PET/CT, to evaluate toxicity and feasibility of high-dose (80 Gy) S-RT. All patients were treated on prostate bed, whereas 20% of patients were treated with additional nodal irradiation. Treatment was generally well tolerated, and no grade 4 toxicity was observed. With a mean follow-up of 31.2 months, the 76.6% of patients were free of recurrence and the 3-year BFS rate was 72.5%.

Despite the good results in terms of BFS showed by the literature, it could be interesting to evaluate even if image-guided S-RT could delay the administration of ADT. ADT still remains the treatment of choice in case of biochemical failure, also after salvage therapies. Nevertheless, hormonal blockade induces several side effects, particularly on the cardiovascular system, and patients eventually progress to castration-resistant prostate cancer.[36]

Berkovic and colleagues[37] investigated whether repeated stereotactic body RT (SBRT) of oligometastatic disease is able to defer the initiation of ADT in patients with low-volume metastases. They enrolled 24 patients with recurrent PCa with up to 3 synchronous metastases (bone and/or LNs) diagnosed on ^{18}F-choline PET/CT, following BR after local curative treatment. Patients were treated with repeated SBRT to a dose of 50 Gy. ADT-free survival defined as the time interval between the first day of SBRT and the initiation of ADT was the primary end point. They concluded that repeated salvage SBRT is feasible, well tolerated, and defers palliative ADT with a median of 38 months in patients with limited bone or LN PCa metastases. **Fig. 1** shows a clinical case of a patient with recurrent PCa who underwent choline PET/CT to restage the disease before S-RT on prostate bed. Considering the detection of PET-positive LNs, S-RT was performed with an enlarged planned target volume and a complete PSA response.

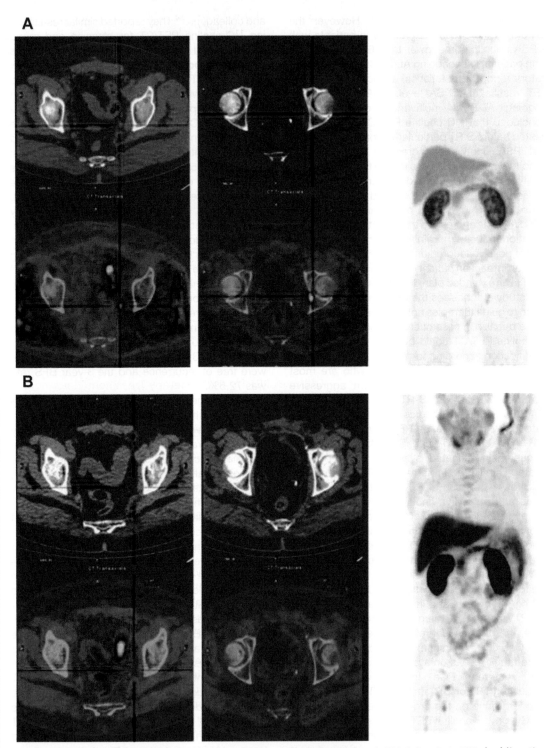

Fig. 1. A 64-year-old patient; RP as primary treatment; T 3a N1 Mx Gs 4 + 4, PSA 2.0 ng/mL, PSA doubling-time 5 months, PSA velocity 1.8 ng/mL/y. (*A*) ^{11}C-choline PET/CT showed the presence of 2 small lesions in the left acebolum and in a small left iliac lymph node. (*B*) ^{11}C-choline PET/CT performed after PET-guided RT: complete response of the lesions. PSA was not measurable at the end of the follow-up Note the presence of few bilateral reactive inguinal lymph nodes.

CHOLINE PET/COMPUTED TOMOGRAPHY TO GUIDE SALVAGE LYMPH NODE DISSECTION

Patients experiencing LN relapse after RP are currently considered as affected by systemic disease and are thus usually addressed to palliative therapies such as ADT. However, evidence exists supporting heterogeneous survival among patients with clinically recurrent PCa.[38,39] In particular, patients with LN relapse showed more favorable outcomes than patients with bone or visceral metastases after radical treatment.[38] In addition, ADT does not represent a potential curative treatment, and many of these patients ultimately develop castration-resistant disease. Moreover, ADT is associated with significant toxicity in the long term.[36] Based on these considerations, PET imaging–guided therapies such as S-PLND have been proposed for patients with LN relapse. Kitajima and colleagues[23] showed a better performance of ^{11}C-choline PET/CT than MR imaging in pelvic lymph node metastasis detection, regardless of PSA values (MR imaging: sensitivity = 64%, specificity = 85%, accuracy = 70%; choline PET: sensitivity = 90%, specificity = 100%, accuracy = 92.9%).

One of the first studies was published by Rinnab and colleagues[40] in a cohort of 15 consecutive patients with increasing PSA values after radical therapy. Patients underwent ^{11}C-choline PET/CT and consecutive open salvage pelvic/retroperitoneal extended LN dissection because of uptake of choline in at least 1 LN. The investigators reported a positive predictive value (PPV) of choline PET of 53%, and generally, S-PLND was well tolerated. More data were provided by Rigatti and colleagues.[41] They reported a biochemical response after salvage surgery in 57% of the enrolled patients (41 of 79 patients), with BFS rates at 3 and 5 year of 27.5% and 10.3%, respectively. The main predictive factors were PSA less than 4 ng/mL at the time of choline PET/CT, time to BR less than 24 months, and negative LNs at the time of RP. Five-year clinical recurrence-free survival was lower for patients with retroperitoneal nodal uptake than for patients with only pelvic positive nodes (11% vs 53%; P<.001). Suardi and colleagues[42] published an update of this study in a subpopulation of this cohort. They evaluated a long follow-up of 8 years and reported a clinical relapse and cancer-specific mortality-free survival rates of 38% and 81%, respectively. On multivariate analysis, PSA at the time of choline PET/CT, biochemical response, and retroperitoneal site of ^{11}C-choline uptake were predictors of earlier clinical relapse. Tilki and colleagues[43] studied 56 patients with PCa showing BR after RP (median

PSA value of 6.0 ng/mL) with ^{18}F-choline PET/CT. After choline PET/CT, all patients underwent bilateral pelvic and/or retroperitoneal lymph adenectomy (1149 LNs were removed). All PET/CT findings were compared with histologic results. The investigators found that 48 of 56 patients (85.7%) with positive ^{18}F-choline PET/CT findings had positive findings on histologic examination. However, on a lesion-based analysis, ^{18}F-choline PET/CT sensitivity, specificity, PPV, and negative predictive value (NPV) were 39.7%, 95.8%, 75.7%, and 83.0%, respectively. A site-based analysis yielded sensitivity, specificity, PPV, and NPV of 68.4%, 73.3%, 81.3%, and 57.9%, respectively. The investigators concluded that a positive ^{18}F-choline PET/CT correctly predicted the presence of LN metastasis in most patients with PCa but did not allow for a precise localization of all metastatic LNs. Passoni and colleagues[44] confirmed these data. They studied 46 patients with BR after RP and a single positive LN at ^{11}C-choline PET/CT. All patients underwent pelvic or pelvic and retroperitoneal LN dissection. Overall, 30 patients (65%) had positive LNs at pathologic examination. ^{11}C-choline PET/CT results were confirmed in 16 patients (35%) who showed pathologically confirmed metastases in the same lymphatic region showed by ^{11}C-choline PET/CT. The overall PPV of ^{11}C-choline PET/CT was 34.8% and 23.9% when exact concordance was defined according to the lymphatic landing site and single positive LN, respectively. The researchers concluded that the poor PPV of ^{11}C-choline PET/CT suggests extensive salvage treatment approaches to maximize the chance of cure.

IMPACT OF PET-GUIDED THERAPIES ON TREATMENT STRATEGY

Considering the new treatment approaches proposed based on choline PET/CT findings, it could be useful to understand if and how PET imaging could influence patient management. Two studies investigated this field to evaluate in which percentage of patients choline PET changed the intended treatment strategy. Soyka and colleagues[45] evaluated retrospectively 156 patients with PCa who had a choline PET/CT performed during BR. The researchers sent questionnaires to the referring physicians after choline PET/CT. Questions included information regarding the scheduled treatment plan before choline PET/CT and the treatment performed after choline PET/CT. Mean follow-up was 42 months. Median PSA values before choline PET/CT and at the end of follow-up were 3.40 ng/mL and 0.91 ng/mL, respectively.

The main finding of the study was that in 75 of the 156 patients (48%), the treatment plan was changed because of the information provided by choline PET/CT. In 33 patients, the therapeutic plan was changed from palliative to curative intent; in 15 patients from curative to palliative, in 8 patients from curative to another strategy, and in 2 patients from one palliative strategy to another. The researchers concluded that choline PET/CT has an important impact on the therapeutic strategy in patients with recurrent PCa and can help to determine an appropriate treatment. Ceci and colleagues[28] enrolled, in a retrospective bicentral trial, 150 patients with recurrent PCa and BR (PSA level, mean 4.3 ng/mL) after radical therapy. Intended treatment before PET/CT was salvage radiotherapy of the prostatic bed in 95 patients and palliative ADT in 55 patients. Effective clinical impact of ^{11}C-choline PET/CT was rated as major (if intended treatment switched from salvage to palliative therapy or vice versa), minor (same treatment, but implemented therapeutic strategy), and none. Mean follow-up was 20.5 months (median 18.3 months, range 6.2–60 months). ^{11}C-choline PET/CT showed positive findings in 109 patients (72.7%), detecting local relapse (prostate bed and/or iliac LNs and/or pararectal LNs) in 64 patients (42.7%). Distant relapse (para-aortic and/or retroperitoneal LNs and/or bone lesions) was seen in 31 patients (20.7%) and both local and distant relapse in 14 (9.3%). Implemented changes of therapy after ^{11}C-choline PET/CT were found in 46.7% (70 of 150) of patients. A major clinical impact was observed in 18% (27 of 150) and a minor clinical impact in 28.7% (43 of 150).

SUMMARY

Despite some limitations mostly due to the suboptimal sensitivity of choline PET/CT, the use of this imaging procedure to guide aggressive therapies in patients with recurrent PCa with an oligometastatic disease is increasing. The detection of few LNs or bone metastasis by PET imaging (oligometastatic patients) should guide the most appropriate treatment instead of palliative systemic therapies. This targeted approach may lead to a better outcome of the patients in terms of BFS and ADT-free survival.

REFERENCES

1. ESMO Guidelines Task Force. ESMO minimum clinical recommendations for diagnosis, treatment and follow-up of prostate cancer. Ann Oncol 2005; 16(suppl 1):i34–6.

2. Heidenreich A, Bastian PJ, Bellmunt J, et al. Guidelines on prostate cancer. Part 1: screening, diagnosis and local treatment with curative intent – update 2013. Eur Urol 2014;65:124–37.

3. Ohori M, Kattan MW, Utsunomiya T, et al. Do impalpable (T1c) cancers visible on ultrasound differ from those not visible? J Urol 2003;169:964–8.

4. Cornud F, Hamida K, Flam T, et al. Endorectal color Doppler sonography and endorectal MR imaging features of nonpalpable prostate cancer: correlation with radical prostatectomy findings. AJR Am J Roentgenol 2000;175:1161–8.

5. Halpern EJ, Frauscher F, Strup SE, et al. Prostate: high-frequency Doppler US imaging for cancer detection. Radiology 2002;225:71–7.

6. Akin O, Sala E, Moskowitz CS, et al. Transition zone prostate cancers: features, detection, localization, and staging at endorectal MR imaging. Radiology 2006;239:784–92.

7. Engelbrecht MR, Huisman HJ, Laheij RJ, et al. Discrimination of prostate cancer from normal peripheral zone and central gland tissue by using dynamic contrast-enhanced MR imaging. Radiology 2003;229:248–54.

8. Buckley DL, Roberts C, Parker GJ, et al. Prostate cancer: evaluation of vascular characteristics with dynamic contrast-enhanced T1-weighted MR imaging—initial experience. Radiology 2004;233:709–15.

9. Ikonen S, Kivisaari L, Vehmas T, et al. Optimal timing of post-biopsy MR imaging of the prostate. Acta Radiol 2001;42:70–3.

10. Qayyum A, Coakley FV, Lu Y, et al. Organ confined prostate cancer: effect of prior transrectal biopsy on endorectal MRI and MR spectroscopic imaging. AJR Am J Roentgenol 2004;183:1079–83.

11. Katz S, Rosen M. MR imaging and MR spectroscopy in prostate cancer management. Radiol Clin North Am 2006;44(5):723–34.

12. Briganti A, Chun FK, Salonia A, et al. Validation of a nomogram predicting the probability of lymph node invasion among patients undergoing radical prostatectomy and an extended pelvic lymphadenectomy. Eur Urol 2006;49(6):1019–26.

13. Freedland SJ, Presti JC Jr, Amling CL, et al. Time trends in biochemical recurrence after radical prostatectomy: results of the SEARCH database. Urology 2003;61:736–41.

14. Hedenreich A, Bastian PJ, Bellmunt J, et al. EAU guidelines on prostate cancer. Part 2: treatment of advanced, relapsing and castration-resistant prostate cancer. Eur Urol 2014;65(2):467–79.

15. Khuntia D, Reddy CA, Mahadevan A, et al. Recurrence-free survival rates after external-beam radiotherapy for patients with clinical T1–T3 prostate carcinoma in the prostate specific antigen era: what should we expect? Cancer 2004; 100:1283–92.

16. Naya Y, Okihara K, Evans RB, et al. Efficacy of prostatic fossa biopsy in detecting local recurrence after radical prostatectomy. Urology 2005;66(2):350–5.

17. Choueiri TK, Dreicer R, Paciorek A, et al. A model that predicts the probability of positive imaging in prostate cancer cases with biochemical failure after initial definitive local therapy J. Urol 2008;179(3):906–10.

18. Phelps ME. Inaugural article: positron emission tomography provides molecular imaging of biological processes. Proc Natl Acad Sci U S A 2000;97:9226–33.

19. Fuccio C, Rubello D, Castellucci P, et al. Choline PET/CT for prostate cancer: main clinical applications. Eur J Radiol 2011;80(2):e50–6.

20. Zeisel SH. Dietary choline: biochemistry, physiology and pharmacology. Annu Rev Nutr 1981;1:95–121.

21. Ackerstaff E, Pflug BR, Nelson JB, et al. Detection of increased choline compounds with proton nuclear magnetic resonance spectroscopy subsequent to malignant transformation of human prostatic epithelial cells. Cancer Res 2001;61:3599–603.

22. Farsad M, Schiavina R, Castellucci P, et al. Detection and localization of prostate cancer: correlation of (11)C-choline PET/CT with histopathologic step-section analysis. J Nucl Med 2005;46:1642–9.

23. Kitajima K, Murphy RC, Nathan MA, et al. Detection of recurrent prostate cancer after radical prostatectomy: comparison of 11C-choline PET/CT with pelvic multiparametric MR imaging with endorectal coil. J Nucl Med 2014;55(2):223–32.

24. Schiavina R, Scattoni V, Castellucci P, et al. (11)C-choline positron emission tomography/computerized tomography for preoperative lymph-node staging in intermediate-risk and high-risk prostate cancer: comparison with clinical staging nomograms. Eur Urol 2008;54:392–401.

25. Punnen S, Cooperberg MR, D'Amico AV, et al. Management of biochemical recurrence after primary treatment of prostate cancer: a systematic review of the literature. Eur Urol 2013;64(6):905–15.

26. Castellucci P, Fuccio C, Nanni C, et al. Influence of trigger PSA and PSA kinetics on ^{11}C-choline PET/CT detection rate in patients with biochemical relapse after radical prostatectomy. J Nucl Med 2009;50:1394–400.

27. Castellucci P, Ceci F, Graziani T, et al. Early biochemical relapse after radical prostatectomy: which prostate cancer patients may benefit from a restaging 11C-choline PET/CT scan before salvage radiation therapy? J Nucl Med 2014;55(9):1424–9.

28. Ceci F, Herrmann K, Castellucci P, et al. Impact of 11C-choline PET/CT on clinical decision making in recurrent prostate cancer: results from a retrospective two-centre trial. Eur J Nucl Med Mol Imaging 2014;41(12):2222–31.

29. Bolla M, Van Tienhoven G, Warde P, et al. External irradiation with or without long-term androgen suppression for prostate cancer with high metastatic risk: 10-year results of an EORTC randomised study. Lancet Oncol 2010;11:1066–73.

30. Stephenson AJ, Scardino PT, Kattan MW, et al. Predicting the outcome of salvage radiation therapy for recurrent prostate cancer after radical prostatectomy. J Clin Oncol 2007;25(15):2035–41.

31. Stephenson AJ, Bolla M, Briganti A, et al. Postoperative radiation therapy for pathologically advanced prostate cancer after radical prostatectomy. Eur Urol 2012;61(3):443–51.

32. Souvatzoglou M, Krause BJ, Pürschel A, et al. Influence of (11)C-choline PET/CT on the treatment planning for salvage radiation therapy in patients with biochemical recurrence of prostate cancer. Radiother Oncol 2011;99(2):193–200.

33. Würschmidt F, Petersen C, Wahl A, et al. [18F]fluoroethylcholine-PET/CT imaging for radiation treatment planning of recurrent and primary prostate cancer with dose escalation to PET/CT-positive lymph nodes. Radiat Oncol 2011;6:44.

34. Picchio M, Berardi G, Fodor A, et al. 11C-choline PET/CT as a guide to radiation treatment planning of lymph-node relapses in prostate cancer patients. Eur J Nucl Med Mol Imaging 2014;41(7):1270–9.

35. D'Angelillo RM, Sciuto R, Ramella S, et al. 18F-choline positron emission tomography/computed tomography-driven high-dose salvage radiation therapy in patients with biochemical progression after radical prostatectomy: feasibility study in 60 patients. Int J Radiat Oncol Biol Phys 2014;90(2):296–302.

36. Schulman C, Irani J, Aapro M. Improving the management of patients with prostate cancer receiving long-term androgen deprivation therapy. BJU Int 2012;109(suppl 6):13–21.

37. Berkovic P, De Meerleer G, Delrue L, et al. Salvage stereotactic body radiotherapy for patients with limited prostate cancer metastases: deferring androgen deprivation therapy. Clin Genitourin Cancer 2013;11(1):27–32.

38. Pond GR, Sonpavde G, de Wit R, et al. The prognostic importance of metastatic site in men with metastatic castration-resistant prostate cancer. Eur Urol 2014;65:3–6.

39. Yossepowitch O, Bianco FJ Jr, Eggener SE, et al. The natural history of noncastrate metastatic prostate cancer after radical prostatectomy. Eur Urol 2007;51:940–8 [discussion: 947–8].

40. Rinnab L, Mottaghy FM, Simon J, et al. [11C]Choline PET/CT for targeted salvage lymph node dissection in patients with biochemical recurrence after primary curative therapy for prostate cancer. Preliminary results of a prospective study. Urol Int 2008;81(2):191–7.

41. Rigatti P, Suardi N, Briganti A, et al. Pelvic/retroperitoneal salvage lymph node dissection for patients

treated with radical prostatectomy with biochemical recurrence and nodal recurrence detected by [11C] choline positron emission tomography/computed tomography. Eur Urol 2011;60(5):935–43.

42. Suardi N, Gandaglia G, Gallina A, et al. Long-term outcomes of salvage lymph node dissection for clinically recurrent prostate cancer: results of a single-institution series with a minimum follow-up of 5 years. Eur Urol 2015;67(2):299–309.

43. Tilki D, Reich O, Graser A, et al. 18F-fluoroethylcholine PET/CT identifies lymph node metastasis in patients with prostate-specific antigen failure after radical prostatectomy but underestimates its extent. Eur Urol 2013;63(5):792–6.

44. Passoni NM, Suardi N, Abdollah F, et al. Utility of [11C]choline PET/CT in guiding lesion-targeted salvage therapies in patients with prostate cancer recurrence localized to a single lymph node at imaging: results from a pathologically validated series. Urol Oncol 2014;32(1):38.e9–16.

45. Soyka JD, Muster MA, Schmid DT, et al. Clinical impact of 18F-choline PET/CT in patients with recurrent prostate cancer. Eur J Nucl Med Mol Imaging 2012;39(6):936–43.

PET/Computed Tomography Using New Radiopharmaceuticals in Targeted Therapy

Punit Sharma, MD, FANMB[a,b], Rakesh Kumar, MD, PhD[b,*], Abass Alavi, MD[c]

KEYWORDS

- PET/CT • Radiopharmaceutical • Targeted therapy • Somatostatin receptor
- Prostate-specific membrane antigen • Hormone receptor • Tyrosine kinase • Angiogenesis

KEY POINTS

- Given the different mechanism of action of targeted therapy compared with conventional chemoradiotherapy, it is often difficult to select suitable patients and monitor therapy response using conventional imaging.
- Molecular PET/computed tomography (CT) imaging with various new radiopharmaceuticals has been evaluated for patient selection and monitoring response to targeted therapy.
- These PET radiopharmaceuticals predominantly target cell surface receptors (surface somatostatin receptor [SSTR], prostate-specific membrane antigen, folate receptor), hormone receptors (estrogen receptor, androgen receptor), receptor tyrosine kinases, or angiogenesis components (vascular endothelial growth factor receptor, integrin $\alpha v \beta 3$).
- Although some of the radiopharmaceuticals (^{68}Ga-SSTR PET/CT) now have established clinical roles, most others are still being evaluated and their exact clinical role is still to be delineated.

TARGETED THERAPY AND PET/COMPUTED TOMOGRAPHY IMAGING

With newer developments in oncologic therapies, there is a new focus on targeted therapies compared with the all-encompassing chemotherapies. These targeted therapies are aimed at various receptors, enzymes, or pathways, and hence are less toxic and more specific than conventional chemoradiotherapies. However, for many targeted agents no predictive biomarkers are available. Molecular imaging with PET can visualize such targets or biochemical processes and/or their dysfunction using specific probes (Fig. 1). In oncology, molecular PET imaging strongly depends on the availability of a specific target on tumor cells or within the tumor stroma or vasculature and the suitability of the designed radiolabeled vector, which depends on its biodistribution, metabolism, affinity, and specificity for the target. Various such radiopharmaceuticals have been developed and explored in the last decade or so. These radiopharmaceuticals help in identification of the presence or absence of various targets in cancer cells for directed therapy, and thus can help in determining the suitability of

Disclosure: The authors have nothing to disclose.
[a] Department of Nuclear Medicine and PET/CT, Eastern Diagnostics India Ltd, 13C Mirza Ghalib Street, Kolkata 700016, India; [b] Diagnostic Nuclear Medicine Division, Department of Nuclear Medicine, All India Institute of Medical Sciences, Ansari Nagar, New Delhi 110029, India; [c] Division of Nuclear Medicine, Department of Radiology, University of Pennsylvania School of Medicine, Hospital of the University of Pennsylvania, 3400 Spruce Street, Philadelphia, PA 19104, USA
* Corresponding author.
E-mail address: rkphulia@yahoo.com

PET Clin 10 (2015) 495–505
http://dx.doi.org/10.1016/j.cpet.2015.05.007

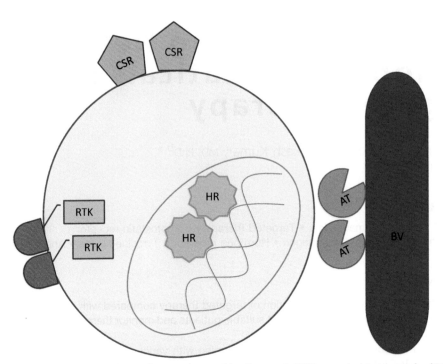

Fig. 1. Cellular and extracellular targets that can be used in diagnostic PET/computed tomography (CT) imaging for targeted therapy. These targets include cell surface receptors (CSR), receptor tyrosine kinase (RTK), intracellular hormonal receptors (HR), and angiogenesis targets (AT) on neo–blood vessels (BV). Various targeted therapies acting on these targets are already available and targeted PET/CT can help in selection of suitable candidates for therapy and response assessment.

patients for targeted therapy with different agents (**Box 1, Table 1**).

PET/COMPUTED TOMOGRAPHY IMAGING OF CELL SURFACE RECEPTORS
Somatostatin Receptors

Structure and expression
Somatostatin receptors (SSTR) are cell surface G-protein–coupled transmembrane receptors that are internalized after binding to a specific ligand.[1] Six such receptors have been identified: SSTR1, SSTR2A, SSTR2B, SSTR3, SSTR4, and SSTR5. Of these, SSTR2 and SSTR5 are predominantly overexpressed in tumors, whereas normal tissue mostly expresses SSTR3 and SSTR5. These

receptors are overexpressed by different cancer cells, including neuroendocrine tumor (NET), paraganglioma, meningioma, and to some extent glioma, breast cancer, head and neck cancer, and lymphoma.[2,3] The SSTR acts as the target for therapy with unlabeled somatostatin (octreotide) and peptide receptor radionuclide therapy (PRRT) with radiolabeled somatostatin analogues.[4,5] Identification of SSTR expression by tumor cells can be assessed by immunohistochemistry (IHC) of a biopsy sample. Given the heterogeneity of SSTR expression by tumors, SSTR-based imaging is a more reproducible and practical method for identifying SSTR expression before targeted therapy.

Somatostatin receptor PET/computed tomography imaging
At present, PET/computed tomography (CT) imaging with ^{68}gallium-1,4,7,10-tetraazacyclododecane-1,4,7,10-tetraacetic acid (^{68}Ga-DOTA) peptides is emerging as the method of choice for SSTR-expressing tumors.[6] These compounds have been shown to have excellent results for diagnosis, staging, restaging, and prognostication of different NETs (**Fig. 2**).[7–9] Three major ^{68}Ga-DOTA peptides are currently available for imaging: ^{68}Ga-DOTA-Phe^1-Tyr^3-octreotide (DOTATOC),

---

Box 1
Therapy targets that have been exploited for PET/CT

- Cell surface receptor
- Hormone receptor
- Receptor tyrosine kinase
- Angiogenesis

Table 1
Brief overview of PET radiopharmaceuticals in targeted therapy

Class	Target	PET Agent	Animal Studies	Human Studies	Clinical Role
Cell surface receptor	Somatostatin receptors	^{68}Ga-DOTATOC	+	+	Established
		^{68}Ga-DOTANOC	+	+	Established
		^{68}Ga-DOTATATE	+	+	Established
		^{64}Cu-DOTATATE	+	+	Under Evaluation
	PSMA	^{68}Ga-PSMA-HBED-CC	+	+	Established
		^{64}Cu-PSMA	+	+	Under Evaluation
		^{18}F-DCFBC	+	+	Under Evaluation
	FR	^{68}Ga-deferoxamine-folate	+	−	Under Evaluation
		^{18}F-fluorobenzylamine-folate	+	−	Under Evaluation
		^{18}F-oligoethyleneglycole-folate	+	−	Under Evaluation
		^{18}F-polyethyleneglycole-folate	+	−	Under Evaluation
Hormone receptor	ER	^{18}F-FES	+	+	Established
	AR	^{18}F-FDHT	+	+	Under Evaluation
Receptor tyrosine kinase	EGFR	^{11}C-erlotinib	+	+	Under Evaluation
		^{11}C-geftinib	+	−	Under Evaluation
		^{18}F-geftinib	+	−	Under Evaluation
		^{64}Cu-cetuximab	+	−	Under Evaluation
		^{86}Y-cetuximab	+	−	Under Evaluation
		^{89}Zr-cetuximab	+	+	Under Evaluation
		^{64}Cu-panitumumab	+	−	Under Evaluation
		^{86}Y-panitumumab	+	−	Under Evaluation
		^{89}Zr-panitumumab	+	−	Under Evaluation
	BCR-ABL	^{11}C-imatinib	−	−	Under Evaluation
	EGFR, HER2	^{18}F-lapatinib	−	−	Under Evaluation
	HER2	^{64}Cu-trastuzumab	+	+	Under Evaluation
		^{89}Zr-trastuzumab	+	+	Under Evaluation
Angiogenesis	VEGFR	^{64}Cu-bevacizumab	+	−	Under Evaluation
		^{86}Y-bevacizumab	+	−	Under Evaluation
		^{89}Zr-bevacizumab	+	+	Under Evaluation
	VEGFR, PDGFR	^{11}C-sorafinib	+	−	Under Evaluation
		^{18}F-sunitinib	−	−	Under Evaluation
		^{11}C-vandetinib	−	−	Under Evaluation
	Integrin αvβ3	^{68}Ga-NODAGA-c(RGDfK)	+	−	Under Evaluation
		^{68}Ga-NOTA-RGD	+	+	Under Evaluation
		^{68}Ga-TRAP (RGD)$_3$	+	−	Under Evaluation
		^{18}F-galacto-RGD	+	−	Under Evaluation
		^{18}F-FPRGD2	+	+	Under Evaluation
		^{18}F-alfatide	+	+	Under Evaluation
		^{64}Cu-NODAGA-c(RGDyK)	−	−	Under Evaluation

Abbreviations: AR, androgen receptor; BCR-ABL, breakpoint cluster region-Abelson murine leukemia viral oncogene; ^{64}Cu-NODAGA-c(RGDfK), ^{64}Cu-1,4,7-triazacyclononane,1-glutaric acid-4,7-acetic acid-cyclo(Arg-Gly-Asp-d-Phe-Lys); DOTANOC, ^{68}Ga-DOTA-Nal^3-octreotide; DOTATATE, ^{68}Ga-DOTA-Tyr^3-octreotate; DOTATOC, ^{68}Ga-DOTA-Phe^1-Tyr^3-octreotide; EGFR, epidermal growth factor receptor; ER, estrogen receptor; ^{18}F-DCFBC, N-[N-[s-1,3-dicarboxypropyl]carbamoyl]-4-^{18}F-fluorobenzyl-L-cysteine; ^{18}F-FDHT, 16β-fluoro-5α-dihyrotestosterone; ^{18}F-FES, 16α-[^{18}F]-fluoro-17β-estradiol; ^{18}F-FPRGD2, ^{18}F-mini-polyethyleneglycol spacered RGD dimer; FR, folate receptor; ^{68}Ga-NODAGA-c(RGDfK), ^{68}Ga-1,4,7-triazacyclononane,1-glutaric acid-4,7-acetic acid-cyclo(Arg-Gly-Asp-d-Phe-Lys); ^{68}Ga-NOTA-RGD, ^{68}Ga-2,2′,2″-(1,4,7-triazonane-1,4,7-triyl)triacetic acid-arginine-glycine-aspartic acid; ^{68}Ga-PSMA-HBED-CC, ^{68}Ga-prostate specific membrane antigen-N,N′-bis-[2-hydroxy-5-(carboxyethyl)benzyl]ethylenediamine-N,N′-diacetic acid; ^{68}Ga-TRAP-(RGD)$_3$, ^{68}Ga-triazacyclononane-phosphinate-(arginine-glycine-aspartic acid)$_3$; HER2, human epidermal growth factor receptor 2; PDGFR, platelet-derived growth factor receptor; PSMA, prostate-specific membrane antigen; VEGFR, vascular endothelial growth factor receptor.

^{68}Ga-DOTA-Nal^3-octreotide (DOTANOC) and ^{68}Ga-DOTA-Tyr^3-Octreotate (DOTATATE). The main difference among these 3 tracers (DOTATOC, DOTANOC, and DOTATATE) is their variable affinity to SSTR subtypes.[10] All of them can bind to SSTR2 and SSTR5, whereas only DOTANOC shows good affinity for SSTR3.[11] The uptake of these ^{68}Ga-DOTA peptides has been proved to

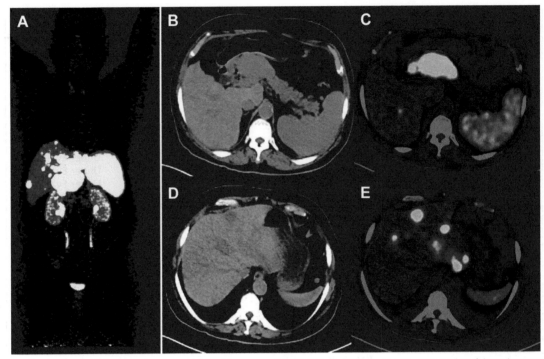

Fig. 2. A 48-year-old man who presented with a mass in the head of pancreas on conventional imaging was referred for PET/CT imaging. ^{68}Ga-DOTA-Nal^3-octreotide (NOC) PET/CT images: whole-body PET projection image showed increased tracer uptake in the region of head of pancreas and liver (*A*). Axial sections of CT and PET/CT confirmed abnormal tracer uptake shown on projection image to be in the head of pancreas and liver (*B–E*). These findings on PET/CT were suggestive of neuroendocrine tumor of head of pancreas with liver metastases.

be directly proportional to SSTR expression by tumor cells, with standardized uptake values (SUVs) correlating with SSTR expression on IHC.[12,13] PET/CT with ^{68}Ga-DOTA peptides has been extensively evaluated for selection of patients for PRRT with ^{177}Lu/^{89}Y-DOTATATE, with the diagnostic-therapeutic pair referred as theranostic twins.[14] Kratochwil and colleagues[15] showed the utility of SUV measured on ^{68}Ga-DOTATOC PET/CT for predicting response to PRRT in metastatic NET, with an SUV value of greater than 16.4 and a tumor/liver ratio of greater than 2.2 predicting response. Ezziddin and colleagues[16] evaluated the relationship between the pretherapeutic tumor SUV in ^{68}Ga-DOTA peptide PET/CT using DOTA-TOC and the mean absorbed tumor dose during subsequent PRRT using ^{177}Lu- DOTATATE. The SUVs were compared with tumor-absorbed doses per injected activity (D/A_0) of the subsequent first treatment cycle. There was a significant correlation between both mean and maximum SUVs, and the D/A_0. The investigators emphasized that, by predicting mean absorbed dose, PET/CT can help in selecting appropriate candidates for PRRT. Also, ^{68}Ga-DOTA peptide PET/CT has been used with success for pretherapy dosimetry of NETs for deciding PRRT dose.[17] The European Neuroendocrine Tumor Society (ENETS) suggests the use of ^{68}Ga-DOTA peptide PET/CT for selection of patients for targeted therapy with PRRT.[18]

Prostate-specific Membrane Antigen

Structure and expression

Prostate-specific membrane antigen (PSMA) is a human transmembrane protein with expression limited to the prostate, the proximal tubules of the kidney, and the brain.[19] The expression is low and isolated in healthy tissues, whereas high-level expression is seen in prostate tumors, especially in metastatic, androgen-independent, and progressive disease (**Figs. 3** and **4**).[20] PSMA is internalized on the binding of certain ligands,[21] providing a mechanism to accumulate PSMA-targeting agents within cells. Recently PSMA has been used a target for targeted radionuclide therapy and immunotherapy for metastatic prostate cancer.[22,23] These developments make PSMA-based PET/CT imaging an important prerequisite.

Prostate-specific membrane antigen PET/computed tomography imaging

In last few years various PET tracers have been developed and evaluated for PSMA-based imaging. Afshar-Oromieh and colleagues[24] evaluated

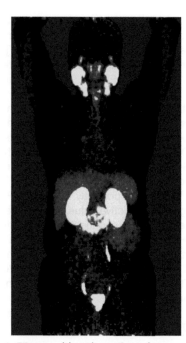

Fig. 3. A 77-year-old male patient, known to have prostate cancer, was referred for ^{68}Ga-PSMA PET/CT for restaging. Whole-body PET projection image showed symmetric increased tracer uptake in salivary glands and proximal gastrointestinal tract (duodenum and jejunum). There is physiologic tracer uptake on ^{68}Ga-PSMA PET/CT.

[68]Ga-Prostate Specific Membrane Antigen-N,N'-bis-[2-hydroxy-5-(carboxyethyl)benzyl]ethylenediamine-N,N'-diacetic acid (^{68}Ga-PSMA-HBED-CC) PET/CT in a large cohort of 319 patients. A lesion-based analysis of sensitivity, specificity, negative predictive value, and positive predictive value revealed values of 76.6%, 100%, 91.4%, and 100%. Demirkol and colleagues[25] showed significant impact of ^{68}Ga-PSMA PET/CT in the management of patients with prostate cancer. Another such compound, ^{68}Ga-PSMA-HBED, has also been successfully evaluated for PET/CT imaging.[26] The ^{18}F-fluoride–labeled tracer N-[N-[s-1,3-dicarboxypropyl]carbamoyl]-4-^{18}F-fluoro-benzyl-L-cysteine (^{18}F-DCFBC), an inhibitor of PSMA, has also been successfully evaluated.[27] Along similar lines, [64]copper (^{64}Cu)-labeled compounds have also been developed for PET imaging.[28] Although still at a nascent stage, PSMA-based PET/CT imaging will most likely develop as an important tool in future for targeted therapy for prostate cancer.

Folate Receptors

Structure and expression
Folate receptors (FRs) are glycoproteins that exist as the isoforms FR-α and FR-β anchored to the cell membrane.[29] Folic acid (or its conjugate) is internalized after binding to FR. FR-α is expressed in renal proximal tubules and in various solid epithelial neoplasms (ovary, endometrium, brain,

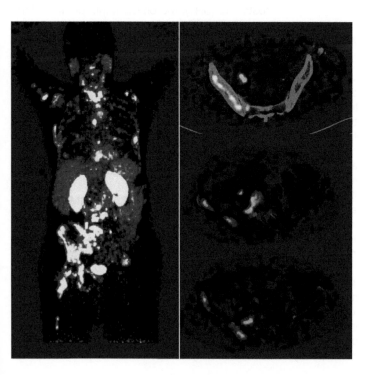

Fig. 4. A 78-year-old male patient, known to have prostate cancer, with increasing prostate-specific antigen level was referred for ^{68}Ga-PSMA PET/CT for restaging. Whole-body PET projection image and multiple PET/CT fused axial images showed focal areas of abnormal increased tracer uptake in multiple bones in the skeleton and multiple pelvic lymph nodes suggestive of metastases.

lung, and renal cancers).[30] FR-β is expressed in normal hematopoietic tissue, activated macrophages, and hematogenous malignancies.[31] Targeting of FR-positive tumor cells in vitro and in vivo has been shown by several research groups using folic acid conjugates with a variety of therapeutic probes.[32] These methods include folic acid–targeted chemotherapeutics,[33] as well as FR-targeted immunotherapy[34] and radionuclide therapy.[35] Thus noninvasive identification of FR on tumor cells is desirable.

Folate receptor PET/computed tomography imaging

Although still investigational, few FR-based PET agents have been evaluated for tumor imaging. Mathias and colleagues[36] reported the radiosynthesis of the first PET folate tracer, ^{68}Ga-deferoxamine folate. FR-positive tumors and kidneys were clearly visualized on small-animal PET images of a tumor-bearing mouse but there was the drawback of a high intestinal accumulation of radioactivity. Various ^{18}F-labeled folate conjugates, such as ^{18}F-fluorobenzylamine-folate[37] and ^{18}F-click folate,[38] have also been synthesized and evaluated. However, because of increased lipophilicity, both tracers had high biliary excretion and intestinal radioactivity. More recently, the new tracers ^{18}F-oligoethyleneglycole folate[39] and ^{18}F-fluoro-polyethyleneglycol (PEG) folate[40] have been synthesized showing reduced lipophilicity. However, in spite of these developments, clinically viable FR PET agents are not yet available.

PET/COMPUTED TOMOGRAPHY IMAGING OF HORMONAL RECEPTOR
Estrogen Receptor

Estrogen receptors (ERs; ERα and ERβ) are intracellular receptors that mediate estrogen signaling and distinctly regulate transcription driving growth, proliferation, and differentiation, among many cellular processes.[41] Apart from normal physiologic function, ERs play an important role in development and progression of various estrogen-dependent cancers (breast, endometrium, and possibly ovaries). Various antiestrogen drugs, such as ER antagonists and aromatase inhibitors, are routinely being used for targeted therapy for these cancers with excellent results.[42] Although tissue biopsy can provide information regarding the primary tumor, in the presence of metastatic disease, targeted imaging with ER agents can provide a whole-body map of ER receptor expression and hence can appropriately guide hormonal therapy versus chemotherapy. This ability is especially important because ER discrepancy

between primary breast cancer and its metastases can be found in up to 40% of patients.[43] Among the ER-based PET agents evaluated, 16α-[^{18}F]-fluoro-17β-estradiol (^{18}F-FES) has been most extensively studied.[44] When ^{18}F-FES PET was compared with the ER expression in tumor biopsies across different studies there was a correlation with a pooled sensitivity of 84% (95% confidence interval [CI], 73%–91%) and a specificity of 98% (95% CI, 90%–100%).[45] In addition, patients with highly ^{18}F-FES–avid lesions were more likely to respond to endocrine therapy than those with low ^{18}F-FES uptake.[46] More importantly, ^{18}F-FES PET has high negative predictive value, thereby helping in the correct selection of patients for endocrine therapies. Heterogeneity of ^{18}F-FES uptake among different lesions can help in individualizing treatment of each lesion.[47,48] To a lesser extent ^{18}F-FES PET has also been evaluated in endometrial[49] and ovarian cancer.[50]

Androgen Receptor

Androgen receptor (AR) is also a cytoplasmic receptor and it plays an important role in development and progression of prostate cancer. Various drugs, including antiandrogens and gonadotropin-releasing hormone analogues, as well as new drugs being evaluated, ultimately act via AR.[51] Hence, PET imaging of AR can help in therapy selection for patients with prostate cancer. 16β-Fluoro-5α-dihyrotestosterone (^{18}F-FDHT) is a structural analogue of 5α-dihydrotestosterone (DHT), the principal intraprostatic form of androgen,[52] and has been extensively evaluated. Dehadashti and colleagues[53] showed a lesion-wise sensitivity of 63% for all lesions and sensitivity of 86% for known lesions for ^{18}F-FDHT PET. Also, treatment with a single dose of the antiandrogen drug flutamide leads to significant reduction in tumor SUV (about 50%). Similar results were also reported by Larson and colleagues.[54] Although further validation is required, ^{18}F-FDHT PET seems to be a promising tracer for guiding AR-targeted prostate cancer therapy.

PET/COMPUTED TOMOGRAPHY IMAGING OF RECEPTOR TYROSINE KINASE
Tyrosine Kinase

Tyrosine kinases (TK) are various enzymes associated with phosphorylation of tyrosine residues of different cellular proteins, leading to a cascade of metabolic events. TK are important clinically because many inhibitors of receptor tyrosine kinases (TKI) have been approved for different cancers. Targeted imaging of TK becomes vital because only a subset of patients show therapeutic response. Various radiolabeled ligands have been developed for PET imaging of receptor TK with PET and could help in choosing therapy. These tracers include radiolabeled natural ligands or their analogues, antibody fragments, affibodies, and nanobodies.[55]

Radiolabeled Drugs or Analogues

Radiolabeled drugs present an important and simple target for TKI PET imaging, because they behave similarly to natural drugs. PET with radiolabeled anticancer drugs provides insight into intratumour drug accumulation as well as target expression. Usually radionuclides are built into the radiotracer. [11]Carbon (^{11}C), or less commonly ^{18}F, is used for radiolabeling these agents. Agents evaluated so far include ^{11}C-erlotinib,[56] ^{11}C-geftinib,[57] ^{18}F-geftinib[58] for epidermal growth factor receptor (EGFR), ^{11}C-imatinib[59] for breakpoint cluster region-Abelson murine leukemia viral oncogene (BCR-ABL) and ^{18}F-lapatinib[60] for both EGFR and human epidermal growth factor receptor 2 (HER2)-related TK. Apart from animal studies, human studies are also available for some of the agents. In one study ^{11}C-erlotinib was shown to be useful for predicting response to erlotinib therapy.[61] Although apparently straightforward, labeled TKIs may form radioactive metabolites that cannot be distinguished from the original drug during PET imaging. This property necessitates direct measurements of the original drug and radiolabeled metabolites in blood samples taken during imaging to accurately quantify drug biodistribution with PET. The position at which radionuclide is added in the molecular structure may influence the formation of radioactive metabolites.

Radiolabeled Antibodies

Different antibodies to different TK receptors are also approved for cancer immunotherapy. These monoclonal antibodies can be labeled and used for imaging. Large sizes of antibodies allow the use of bifunctional chelates (DOTA, NOTA, desferrioxamine).[62] Radiolabeled antibodies have slow kinetics and target binding, which necessitates delayed PET imaging. Hence, such tracers are labeled with PET radionuclides with long half-lives, such as ^{64}Cu, [89]Zr, and [86]Y. PET agents that have been evaluated for this purpose include ^{64}Cu/[89]Zr-trastuzumab[63,64] for HER2, and ^{64}Cu/[86]Y/[89]Zr-cetuximab[65–67] and ^{64}Cu/[86]Y/[89]Zr-panitumumab[68–70] for EGFR TK. Mortimer and colleagues[71] showed the utility of ^{64}Cu-DOTA-trastuzumab PET in noninvasive whole-body mapping of HER2-positive lesions in patients with metastatic breast cancer. Similarly, Gootjes and colleagues[72] showed the utility of [89]Zr-cetuximab-PET imaging for EGFR mapping in metastatic colon cancer. Given the large size of monoclonal antibodies, various researchers have also evaluated antibody fragments and affibodies.[73]

PET/COMPUTED TOMOGRAPHY IMAGING OF ANGIOGENESIS
Target and Expression

Angiogenesis plays an important role in sustenance and progression of solid tumors. Hence, drugs targeting angiogenesis are being used in different cancers (eg, bevacizumab, sorafenib, everolimus). Targeted PET imaging for angiogenesis can help in identifying patients who will respond to these drugs and also for response monitoring. The two major targets for PET angiogenesis imaging are vascular endothelial growth factor receptor (VEGFR) and integrin $\alpha v \beta 3$.[74] Vascular endothelial growth factor (VEGF) is the most significant and potent stimulator of angiogenesis. VEGF ligands, of which there are 4 known isoforms, mediate their angiogenic effects by binding to specific receptors (VEGFR1– VEGFR3), leading to receptor dimerization and subsequent intracellular signal transduction via TK.[75] In contrast, integrin $\alpha v \beta 3$, a heterodimeric cell surface receptor, plays a significant role in angiogenesis by allowing cells to interact with the extracellular matrix, contributing to the migration of endothelial cells.[76]

PET/Computed Tomography Imaging

Three categories of PET agents have been evaluated for angiogenesis imaging: radiolabeled antibodies, radiolabeled drugs, and radiolabeled peptidomimetics such as RGD (arginine-glycine-aspartate).[77] [64]Cu/[86]Y/[89]Zr-bevacizumab has been studied for PET angiogenesis imaging.[78–80] These agents have also been evaluated for monitoring response to antiangiogenic agents.[81,82] Radiolabeled antiangiogenic drugs such as ^{11}C-sorafinib,[83] ^{18}F-sunitinib,[84] and ^{11}C-vanetinib[85] have also been evaluated for PET angiogenesis imaging, although in few animal studies. Use of radiolabeled peptidomimetics such as RGD has been extensively evaluated, especially because of the ease of labeling using bifunctional chelates. The RGD peptides have very high affinity for integrin $\alpha v \beta 3$. Different RGD peptides have been labeled with ^{68}Ga, ^{18}F, and ^{64}Cu and used for PET imaging.[86] Withofs and colleagues[87] showed the utility of ^{18}F-mini-PEG spacered RGD dimer (^{18}F-FPRGD2) for angiogenesis imaging in patients with renal cell carcinoma, but the utility was limited to non–$\alpha v \beta 3$-expressing tumors. Various 68Ga-labeled tracers are now being actively evaluated. One such tracer, ^{68}Ga-1,4,7-triazacyclononane,1-glutaric acid-4,7-acetic acid-cyclo(Arg-Gly-Asp-d-Phe-Lys) [^{68}Ga-NO-DAGA-c(RGDfK)], is being actively pursued as a potential theranostic agent.[88] However, successful antiangiogenic therapy with bevacizumab did not show any appreciable change in ^{68}Ga-NODAGA-c(RGDfK) uptake on PET.[89] Other tracers evaluated for this purpose include ^{18}F-galacto-RGD, ^{18}F-alfatide, ^{68}Ga-2,2',2"-(1,4,7-triazonane-1,4,7-triyl) triacetic acid-arginine-glycine-aspartic acid (^{68}Ga-NOTA-RGD), ^{68}Ga-triazacyclononane-phosphinate-(arginine-glycine-aspartic acid)$_3$ [^{68}Ga-TRAP-(RGD)$_3$], and ^{64}Cu-1,4,7-triazacyclo-nonane,1-glutaric acid-4,7-acetic acid-cyclo(Arg-Gly-Asp-d-Phe-Lys) [^{64}Cu-NODAGA-c(RGDfK)].[90] Further research in this field is warranted.

REFERENCES

1. Cescato R, Schulz S, Waser B, et al. Internalization of sst2, sst3, and sst5 receptors: effects of somatostatin agonists and antagonists. J Nucl Med 2006; 47:502–11.

2. de Herder WW, Hofland LJ, van der Lely AJ, et al. Somatostatin receptors in gastroentero-pancreatic neuroendocrine tumours. Endocr Relat Cancer 2003;10:451–8.

3. Frati A, Rouzier R, Lesieur B, et al. Expression of somatostatin type-2 and -4 receptor and correlation with histological type in breast cancer. Anticancer Res 2014;34:3997–4003.

4. Kwekkeboom DJ, Krenning EP, Lebtahi R, et al. ENETS consensus guidelines for the standards of care in neuroendocrine tumors: peptide receptor radionuclide therapy with radiolabeled somatostatin analogs. Neuroendocrinology 2009;90:220–6.

5. Van Essen M, Krenning EP, De Jong M, et al. Peptide receptor radionuclide therapy with radiolabelled somatostatin analogues in patients with somatostatin receptor positive tumours. Acta Oncol 2007; 46:723–34.

6. Sharma P, Singh H, Bal C, et al. PET/CT imaging of neuroendocrine tumors with (68)gallium-labeled somatostatin analogues: an overview and single institutional experience from India. Indian J Nucl Med 2014;29:2–12.

7. Naswa N, Sharma P, Kumar A, et al. Gallium-68-DOTA-NOC PET/CT of patients with gastroentero-pancreatic neuroendocrine tumors: a prospective single-center study. AJR Am J Roentgenol 2011; 197:1221–8.

8. Sharma P, Dhull VS, Arora S, et al. Diagnostic accuracy of (68)Ga-DOTANOC PET/CT imaging in pheochromocytoma. Eur J Nucl Med Mol Imaging 2014; 41:494–504.

9. Sharma P, Naswa N, Kc SS, et al. Comparison of the prognostic values of 68Ga-DOTANOC PET/CT and 18F-FDG PET/CT in patients with well-differentiated neuroendocrine tumor. Eur J Nucl Med Mol Imaging 2014;41:2194–202.

10. Antunes P, Ginj M, Zhang H, et al. Are radiogallium-labelled DOTA-conjugated somatostatin analogues superior to those labelled with other radiometals? Eur J Nucl Med Mol Imaging 2007;34:982–93.

11. Wild D, Mäcke HR, Waser B, et al. 68Ga-DOTANOC: a first compound for PET imaging with high affinity for somatostatin receptor subtypes 2 and 5. Eur J Nucl Med Mol Imaging 2005;32:724.

12. Miederer M, Seidl S, Buck A, et al. Correlation of immunohistopathological expression of somatostatin receptor 2 with standardised uptake values in 68Ga-DOTATOC PET/CT. Eur J Nucl Med Mol Imaging 2009;36:48–52.

13. Kaemmerer D, Peter L, Lupp A, et al. Molecular imaging with ^{68}Ga-SSTR PET/CT and correlation to immunohistochemistry of somatostatin receptors in neuroendocrine tumours. Eur J Nucl Med Mol Imaging 2011;38:1659–68.

14. Werner RA, Bluemel C, Allen-Auerbach MS, et al. (68)Gallium- and (90)yttrium-/(177)lutetium: "theranostic twins" for diagnosis and treatment of NETs. Ann Nucl Med 2015;29:1–7.

15. Kratochwil C, Stefanova M, Mavriopoulou E, et al. SUV of [68Ga]DOTATOC-PET/CT predicts response probability of PRRT in neuroendocrine tumors. Mol Imaging Biol 2015;17(3):313–8.

16. Ezziddin S, Lohmar J, Yong-Hing CJ, et al. Does the pretherapeutic tumor SUV in 68Ga DOTATOC PET predict the absorbed dose of 177Lu octreotate? Clin Nucl Med 2012;37:e141–7.

17. Blaickner M, Baum RP. Relevance of PET for pretherapeutic prediction of doses in peptide receptor radionuclide therapy. PET Clin 2014;9:99–112.

18. Baum RP, Kulkarni HR. THERANOSTICS: from molecular imaging using Ga-68 labeled tracers and PET/CT to personalized radionuclide therapy - the Bad Berka experience. Theranostics 2012;2: 437–47.

19. Rajasekaran AK, Anilkumar G, Christiansen JJ. Is prostate-specific membrane antigen a multifunctional protein? Am J Physiol Cell Physiol 2005;288: C975–81.

20. Barrett JA, Coleman RE, Goldsmith SJ, et al. First-in-man evaluation of 2 high-affinity PSMA-avid small molecules for imaging prostate cancer. J Nucl Med 2013;54:380–7.

21. Liu H, Rajasekaran AK, Moy P, et al. Constitutive and antibody-induced internalization of prostate-specific membrane antigen. Cancer Res 1998;58:4055–60.

22. Santoni M, Scarpelli M, Mazzucchelli R, et al. Targeting prostate-specific membrane antigen for personalized therapies in prostate cancer: morphologic

and molecular backgrounds and future promises. J Biol Regul Homeost Agents 2014;28:555–63.

23. Tagawa ST, Milowsky MI, Morris M, et al. Phase II study of lutetium-177-labeled anti-prostate-specific membrane antigen monoclonal antibody J591 for metastatic castration-resistant prostate cancer. Clin Cancer Res 2013;19:5182–91.

24. Afshar-Oromieh A, Avtzi E, Giesel FL, et al. The diagnostic value of PET/CT imaging with the (68)Ga-labelled PSMA ligand HBED-CC in the diagnosis of recurrent prostate cancer. Eur J Nucl Med Mol Imaging 2015;42:197–209.

25. Demirkol MO, Acar Ö, Uçar B, et al. Prostate-specific membrane antigen-based imaging in prostate cancer: impact on clinical decision making process. Prostate 2015;75(7):748–57.

26. Krohn T, Verburg FA, Pufe T, et al. [(68)Ga]PSMA-HBED uptake mimicking lymph node metastasis in coeliac ganglia: an important pitfall in clinical practice. Eur J Nucl Med Mol Imaging 2015;42:210–4.

27. Cho SY, Gage KL, Mease RC, et al. Biodistribution, tumor detection, and radiation dosimetry of 18F-DCFBC, a low-molecular-weight inhibitor of prostate-specific membrane antigen, in patients with metastatic prostate cancer. J Nucl Med 2012; 53:1883–91.

28. Banerjee SR, Pullambhatla M, Foss CA, et al. ^{64}Cu-labeled inhibitors of prostate-specific membrane antigen for PET imaging of prostate cancer. J Med Chem 2014;57:2657–69.

29. Elnakat H, Ratnam M. Distribution, functionality and gene regulation of folate receptor isoforms: implications in targeted therapy. Adv Drug Deliv Rev 2004; 56:1067–84.

30. Parker N, Turk MJ, Westrick E, et al. Folate receptor expression in carcinomas and normal tissues determined by a quantitative radioligand binding assay. Anal Biochem 2005;338:284–93.

31. Reddy JA, Haneline LS, Srour EF, et al. Expression and functional characterization of the β-isoform of the folate receptor on CD34+ cells. Blood 1999;93:3940–8.

32. Zhao X, Li H, Lee RJ. Targeted drug delivery via folate receptors. Expert Opin Drug Deliv 2008;5: 309–19.

33. Li J, Sausville EA, Klein PJ, et al. Clinical pharmacokinetics and exposure-toxicity relationship of a folate-Vinca alkaloid conjugate EC145 in cancer patients. J Clin Pharmacol 2009;49:1467–76.

34. Lu Y, Sega E, Leamon CP, et al. Folate receptor-targeted immunotherapy of cancer: mechanism and therapeutic potential. Adv Drug Deliv Rev 2004;56:1161–76.

35. Müller C, Schibli R. Prospects in folate receptor-targeted radionuclide therapy. Front Oncol 2013; 3:249.

36. Mathias CJ, Lewis MR, Reichert DE, et al. Preparation of 66Ga- and 68Ga-labeled Ga(III)-

deferoxamine-folate as potential folate-receptor-targeted PET radiopharmaceuticals. Nucl Med Biol 2003;30:725–31.

37. Bettio A, Honer M, Müller C, et al. Synthesis and preclinical evaluation of a folic acid derivative labeled with 18F for PET imaging of folate receptor-positive tumors. J Nucl Med 2006;47:1153–60.

38. Ross TL, Honer M, Lam PY, et al. Fluorine-18 click radiosynthesis and preclinical evaluation of a new 18F-labeled folic acid derivative. Bioconjug Chem 2008;19:2462–70.

39. Schieferstein H, Betzel T, Fischer CR, et al. 18 F-click labeling and preclinical evaluation of a new 18 F-folate for PET imaging. EJNMMI Res 2013;3:68.

40. Gent YJ, Weijers K, Molthoff CF, et al. Evaluation of the novel folate receptor ligand [18F]fluoro-PEG-folate for macrophage targeting in a rat model of arthritis. Arthritis Res Ther 2013;15:R37.

41. Shao W, Brown M. Advances in estrogen receptor biology: prospects for improvements in targeted breast cancer therapy. Breast Cancer Res 2004;6: 39–52.

42. Shanle EK, Xu W. Selectively targeting estrogen receptors for cancer treatment. Adv Drug Deliv Rev 2010;62:1265–76.

43. Amir E, Clemons M, Purdie CA. Tissue confirmation of disease recurrence in breast cancer patients: pooled analysis of multi-centre, multi-disciplinary prospective studies. Cancer Treat Rev 2012;38: 708–14.

44. Mankoff DA, Link JM, Linden HM, et al. Tumor receptor imaging. J Nucl Med 2008;49:149S–63S.

45. van Kruchten M, de Vries EG, de Vries EF, et al. PET imaging of oestrogen receptors in patients with breast cancer. Lancet Oncol 2013;14:e465–75.

46. Dehdashti F, Mortimer JE, Trinkaus K, et al. PET-based estradiol challenge as a predictive biomarker of response to endocrine therapy in women with estrogen-receptor-positive breast cancer. Breast Cancer Res Treat 2009;113:509–17.

47. Sun Y, Yang Z, Zhang Y, et al. The preliminary study of 16α-[18F]fluoroestradiol PET/CT in assisting the individualized treatment decisions of breast cancer patients. PLoS One 2015;10:e0116341.

48. Dixit M, Shi J, Wei L, et al. Synthesis of clinical-grade [18F]-fluoroestradiol as a surrogate PET biomarker for the evaluation of estrogen receptor-targeting therapeutic drug. Int J Mol Imaging 2013;2013: 278607.

49. Tsujikawa T, Yoshida Y, Maeda H, et al. Oestrogen-related tumour phenotype: positron emission tomography characterisation with 18F-FDG and 18F-FES. Br J Radiol 2012;85:1020–4.

50. Yoshida Y, Kurokawa T, Tsujikawa T, et al. Positron emission tomography in ovarian cancer: 18F-deoxy-glucose and 16α-18F-fluoro-17β-estradiol PET. J Ovarian Res 2009;2:7.

51. Chen Y, Clegg NJ, Scher HI. Antiandrogens and androgen depleting therapies in prostate cancer: novel agents for an established target. Lancet Oncol 2009;10:981–91.

52. Choe YS, Lidström PJ, Chi DY, et al. Synthesis of 11 beta-[18F]fluoro-5 alpha-dihydrotestosterone and 11 beta-[18F]fluoro-19-nor-5 alpha-dihydrotestosterone: preparation via halofluorination-reduction, receptor binding, and tissue distribution. J Med Chem 1995;38:816–25.

53. Dehdashti F, Picus J, Michalski JM, et al. Positron tomographic assessment of androgen receptors in prostatic carcinoma. Eur J Nucl Med Mol Imaging 2005;32:344–50.

54. Larson SM, Morris M, Gunther I, et al. Tumor localization of 16beta-18F-fluoro-5alpha-dihydrotestosterone versus 18F-FDG in patients with progressive, metastatic prostate cancer. J Nucl Med 2004;45: 366–73.

55. Mammatas LH, Verheul HM, Hendrikse NH, et al. Molecular imaging of targeted therapies with positron emission tomography: the visualization of personalized cancer care. Cell Oncol (Dordr) 2015; 38:49–64.

56. Bahce I, Smit EF, Lubberink M, et al. Development of [11C]erlotinib positron emission tomography for in vivo evaluation of EGF receptor mutational status. Clin Cancer Res 2013;19:183–93.

57. Zhang MR, Kumata K, Hatori A, et al. [11C]Gefitinib ([11c]Iressa): radiosynthesis, in vitro uptake, and in vivo imaging of intact murine fibrosarcoma. Mol Imaging Biol 2010;12:181–91.

58. Su H, Seimbille Y, Ferl GZ, et al. Evaluation of [18F] gefitinib as a molecular imaging probe for the assessment of the epidermal growth factor receptor status in malignant tumors. Eur J Nucl Med Mol Imaging 2008;35:1089–99.

59. Kil KE, Ding YS, Lin KS, et al. Synthesis and positron emission tomography studies of carbon-11-labeled imatinib (Gleevec). Nucl Med Biol 2007;34:153–63.

60. Basuli F, Wu H, Li C, et al. A first synthesis of 18F-radiolabeled lapatinib: a potential tracer for positron emission tomographic imaging of ErbB1/ErbB2 tyrosine kinase activity. J Labelled Comp Radiopharm 2011;54:633–6.

61. Memon AA, Weber B, Winterdahl M, et al. PET imaging of patients with non-small cell lung cancer employing an EGF receptor targeting drug as tracer. Br J Cancer 2011;6(105):1850–5.

62. Brechbiel MW. Bifunctional chelates for metal nuclides. Q J Nucl Med Mol Imaging 2008;52:166–73.

63. Tamura K, Kurihara H, Yonemori K, et al. 64Cu-DOTA-trastuzumab PET imaging in patients with HER2-positive breast cancer. J Nucl Med 2013;51:1869–75.

64. Dijkers EC, Munnink TH, Kosterink JG, et al. Biodistribution of 89Zr-trastuzumab and PET imaging

of HER2-positive lesions in patients with metastatic breast cancer. Clin Pharmacol Ther 2010;87:586–92.

65. Achmad A, Hanaoka H, Yoshioka H, et al. Predicting cetuximab accumulation in KRAS wild-type and KRAS mutant colorectal cancer using 64Cu-labeled cetuximab positron emission tomography. Cancer Sci 2012;103:600–5.

66. Nayak TK, Garmestani K, Milenic DE, et al. HER1-targeted 86Y-panitumumab possesses superior targeting characteristics than 86Y-cetuximab for PET imaging of human malignant mesothelioma tumors xenografts. PLoS One 2011;25:101371.

67. Perk LR, Visser GW, Vosjan MJ, et al. (89)Zr as a PET surrogate radioisotope for scouting biodistribution of the therapeutic radiometals (90)Y and (177)Lu in tumor-bearing nude mice after coupling to the internalizing antibody cetuximab. J Nucl Med 2005;46:1898–906.

68. Niu G, Li Z, Xie J, et al. PET of EGFR antibody distribution in head and neck squamous cell carcinoma models. J Nucl Med 2009;50:1116–23.

69. Nayak TK, Garmestani K, Baidoo KE, et al. Preparation, biological evaluation, and pharmacokinetics of the human anti-HER1 monoclonal antibody panitumumab labeled with 86Y for quantitative PET of carcinoma. J Nucl Med 2010;51:942–50.

70. Chang AJ, De Silva RA, Lapi SE. PET and MRI of metastatic peritoneal and pulmonary colorectal cancer in mice with human epidermal growth factor receptor 1-targeted 89Zr-labeled panitumumab. Mol Imaging 2013;12:17–27.

71. Mortimer JE, Bading JR, Colcher DM, et al. Functional imaging of HER2-positive metastatic breast cancer using 64Cu-DOTA-trastuzumab positron emission tomography. J Nucl Med 2014;55:23–9.

72. Gootjes EC, Huisman MC, Vughts D, et al. [89Zr] labeled cetuximab PET imaging in advanced colorectal cancer patients: a feasibility study. Abstract O3.6 of the 12th international congress on targeted anticancer therapies 2014. Available at: http://www.tatcongress.org/previous-tatcongresses/tat-2014/download-abstracts/. Accessed April 18, 2014.

73. Beylergil V, Morris PG, Smith-Jones PM, et al. Pilot study of 68Ga-DOTA-F(ab')2-trastuzumab in patients with breast cancer. Nucl Med Commun 2013; 34:1157–65.

74. Lu X, Wang RF. A concise review of current radiopharmaceuticals in tumor angiogenesis imaging. Curr Pharm Des 2012;18:1032–40.

75. Bruce D, Tan PH. Vascular endothelial growth factor receptors and the therapeutic targeting of angiogenesis in cancer: where do we go from here? Cell Commun Adhes 2011;18:85–103.

76. Brooks PC, Clark RA, Cheresh DA. Requirement of vascular integrin alpha v beta 3 for angiogenesis. Science 1994;264:569–71.

77. Stacy MR, Maxfield MW, Sinusas AJ. Targeted molecular imaging of angiogenesis in PET and SPECT: a review. Yale J Biol Med 2012;85:75–86.

78. Paudyal B, Paudyal P, Oriuchi N, et al. Positron emission tomography imaging and biodistribution of vascular endothelial growth factor with 64Cu-labeled bevacizumab in colorectal cancer xenografts. Cancer Sci 2011;102:117–21.

79. Nayak TK, Garmestani K, Baidoo KE, et al. PET imaging of tumor angiogenesis in mice with VEGF-A-targeted (86)Y-CHX-A''-DTPA-bevacizumab. Int J Cancer 2011;128:920–6.

80. van der Bilt AR, van Scheltinga ATG, Timmer-Bosscha H, et al. Measurement of tumor VEGF-A levels with 89Zr-bevacizumab PET as an early biomarker for the antiangiogenic effect of everolimus treatment in an ovarian cancer xenograft model. Clin Cancer Res 2012;18:6306–14.

81. Oosting S, Brouwers AH, van Es SC, et al. 89Zr-bevacizumab PET imaging in metastatic renal cell carcinoma patients before and during antiangiogenic treatment. J Clin Oncol 2012;30(suppl 15):10581.

82. Chang AJ, Sohn R, Lu ZH, et al. Detection of rapalog-mediated therapeutic response in renal cancer xenografts using 64Cu-bevacizumab immunoPET. PLoS One 2013;8:101371.

83. Asakawa C, Ogawa M, Kumata K, et al. [11C]Sorafenib: radiosynthesis and preliminary PET study of brain uptake in P-gp/Bcrp knockout mice. Bioorg Med Chem Lett 2011;21:2220–3.

84. Wang JQ, Miller KD, Sledge GW, et al. Synthesis of [18F]SU11248, a new potential PET tracer for imaging cancer tyrosine kinase. Bioorg Med Chem Lett 2005;15:4380–4.

85. Gao M, Lola CM, Wang M, et al. Radiosynthesis of [11C]vandetanib and [11C]chloro-vandetanib as new potential PET agents for imaging of VEGFR in cancer. Bioorg Med Chem Lett 2011;21:3222–6.

86. Tateishi U, Oka T, Inoue T. Radiolabeled RGD peptides as integrin alpha(v)beta3-targeted PET tracers. Curr Med Chem 2012;19:3301–9.

87. Withofs N, Signolle N, Somja J, et al. 18F-FPRGD2 PET/CT imaging of integrin αvβ3 in renal carcinomas: correlation with histopathology. J Nucl Med 2015;56(3):361–4.

88. Lopez-Rodriguez V, Gaspar-Carcamo RE, Pedraza-Lopez M, et al. Preparation and preclinical evaluation of (66)Ga-DOTA-E(c(RGDfK))2 as a potential theranostic radiopharmaceutical. Nucl Med Biol 2015;42:109–14.

89. Rylova SN, Barnucz E, Fani M, et al. Does imaging αvβ3 integrin expression with PET detect changes in angiogenesis during bevacizumab therapy? J Nucl Med 2014;55:1878–84.

90. Haubner R, Maschauer S, Prante O. PET radiopharmaceuticals for imaging integrin expression: tracers in clinical studies and recent developments. Biomed Res Int 2014;2014:871609.

PET/Computed Tomography in Evaluation of Transarterial Chemoembolization

Nayelli Ortega López, MD[a,b,*]

KEYWORDS

- ^{18}F-FDG • PET/CT • HCC • TACE • Treatment response

KEY POINTS

- Transarterial chemoembolization (TACE) is a minimally invasive procedure that deprives the tumor of its blood supply, and is especially used for the treatment of unresectable hepatocellular carcinoma.
- One approach used to accurately evaluate tumor viability before retreatment, either by surgery or by repeated TACE, is ^{18}F-fluorodeoxyglucose PET.
- The most useful imaging modality for identifying viable tumor versus tumor necrosis is PET, which provides in vivo metabolic information.

INTRODUCTION

Hepatocellular carcinoma (HCC) is one of the most common cancers worldwide, being the sixth most common cancer and the third leading cause of cancer-related death worldwide.[1]

Future incidences and mortalities for HCC are projected to largely increase in several regions around the world, mostly as a result of the dissemination of hepatitis C virus infection. For this reason, surveillance programs have been implemented for cirrhotic patients.

However, approximately 70% to 80% of patients with HCC cannot receive curative treatments such as surgical resection (SR), liver transplantation (LT), or ablative therapies because diagnosis is usually made at an intermediate to advanced stage of the disease, which is too late for patients to endure the surgical insults, especially if associated liver cirrhosis conditions have caused a poor liver functional reserve.[1–3]

Also, in a high proportion of cases the disease recurs after attempts at curative therapy. For these reasons, the prognosis of patients with HCC remains poor, and life expectancy is difficult to predict because of variable factors that include aggressiveness of the tumor, metabolic change, tumor burden, and liver reserve function.[2]

Palliative therapies for patients with inoperative HCC include transarterial chemoembolization (TACE), systemic chemotherapy, radiofrequency thermal ablation therapy, radioembolization, local injection therapy, and immunotherapy. TACE is an effective curative or palliative treatment with a significant survival benefit for intermediate HCC[1,4]; however, the literature reports a high incidence of

Disclosure: The author has nothing to disclose.
[a] Department of Nuclear Medicine, Instituto Nacional de Cancerología, Av. San Fernando, no. 22, Colonia Sección XVI, C.P. 0400, Mexico City, Mexico; [b] PET/CT Unit, Imagenus, Advanced Diagnostics in Healthcare, Av. México-Coyoacán, no. 346, Colonia General Anaya, Mexico City 03340, Mexico
* PET/CT Unit, Imagenus. Av. México-Coyoacán, no. 346, Colonia General Anaya, Ciudad de México 03340, México.
E-mail address: nayeortega2000@yahoo.com.mx

tumor recurrence, with rates approximately of 22.3% at 6 months and 78% at 12 months.[3]

It is therefore important to accurately evaluate tumor viability before retreatment, either by surgery or by repeated TACE. One approach used to assess the biological activity of a tumor is PET.

TRANSARTERIAL CHEMOEMBOLIZATION DEFINITION AND TYPES

The success of TACE results from the current knowledge of the hepatic circulation and the advances in interventional radiology. Eighty percent of the blood supply in the normal liver is from the portal vein and the rest is from the hepatic artery but, in neoplastic tissue, the hepatic artery supplies almost 100% of the nutrients.[4] TACE differs from transcatheter arterial embolization because the latter does not allow anticancer drug administration.

TACE is a minimally invasive procedure, the objective of which is to deprive the tumor of its blood supply by injecting embolic agents into the tumor-feeding artery for a successful vessel obstruction after administering a sustained concentration of high doses of chemotherapy, resulting in a strong cytotoxic effect enhanced by ischemic necrosis of the targeted tumor.[1,4–6] The benefit of this technique is that the chemotherapeutic drug is not washed out from the vascular bed by blood flow after embolization.

Since its introduction in 1974 by Doyon and colleagues[7] for the treatment of unresectable HCC, TACE has undergone several developments, such as the use of lipiodol (mid-1990s), which mainly enhanced the therapeutic effect by acting as a drug carrier, retaining the anticancer drug for a longer period of time in the tumor (several weeks compared with around 7 days in normal liver) and increasing the cytotoxic effect.[4,8,9]

In general, the conventional TACE (cTACE) technique consists of the intra-arterial injection of a viscous emulsion, consisting of a chemotherapeutic drug such as doxorubicin or cisplatin mixed with iodized oil or lipiodol, followed by embolization of the tumor-feeding artery with either a spherical or a nonspherical embolic agent (usually gelatin sponge particles).

The embolization end point is usually defined as stasis in the second-order or third-order branches of the lobar hepatic artery.[5] Liver functional reserve is a critical component for careful patient selection for TACE, because the ischemic insult can lead to severe adverse events, being absolutely contraindicated in patients with decompensated liver cirrhosis or Child-Pugh C, severely reduced portal vein flow caused by nontumoral portal vein occlusion or a large arterioportal shunt, massive invasion of both lobes, extrahepatic spread or involvement of the major branches of the portal vein or the portal trunk, or renal deficiency.[1,4]

This invasive technique has become the standard treatment of patients with intermediate-stage HCC according to the Barcelona Clinic Liver Cancer (BCLC-B) staging system, or patients with Child-Pugh A or B without ascites and with multiple HCCs (European Association for the Study of the Liver [EASL]) who are not eligible for surgical resection (large or multinodular HCC and preserved liver function, absence of cancer-related symptoms, and no evidence of vascular invasion or extrahepatic spread).

TACE is also proposed as an alternative to surgery in early stage HCC, as preoperative (SR or LT) adjuvant chemotherapy in patients with liver tumors with the aim of downstaging the lesion before surgery and improving survival, in patients with regional recurrence of HCC after previous resection, in cholangiocarcinoma, in some neuroendocrine tumors, sarcomas, and in liver-dominant metastases from other primary malignancies and uveal melanoma.[10–12]

Superselective TACE is a variant of TACE designed for the embolization of the distal portion of the feeding subsegmental hepatic artery to induce sever ischemic effects on a small area of the liver, with the subsequent reduction of liver damage and adverse events. Several experts have reported complete tumor necrosis in tumors sized less than 4 to 5 cm in 40% to 70% of patients with HCC, or patients who remain local tumor progression free for more than 3 years.[4]

However, the absence of global guidelines with regard to optimal chemotherapeutic agents dose and the choice or combination of cytotoxic agents for TACE, as well as the variability in the performance of this technique, results in difficulties in comparing the data between different TACE studies.[4] Some other options have been developed offering a more standardized approach to HCC treatment, with higher levels of consistency and repeatability compared with cTACE, as well as similar response rates to Gelfoam-lipiodol particles, and fewer systemic adverse effects, such as embolic drug-eluting bead (DEB) TACE with doxorubicin or epirubicin (DEB-TACE). In Japan, mitomycin, cisplatin, and miriplatin have also been used for this technique, but there is also no consensus on the optimal chemotherapeutic agents to use.[4,11,13] This treatment modality ensures sustained and slow release of the chemotherapeutic drug locally in addition to causing ischemic injury to the tumor and it has been shown that DEB-TACE can result in an overall favorable toxicity profile and anticancer efficacy, with higher rates of complete response, objective response (OR), and disease control than cTACE.[14]

Several studies, including randomized controlled trials (RCTs), have shown the significantly reduced liver toxicity and the safe pharmacokinetic profile, as well as the longer time to progression (TTP), of DEB-TACE loaded with doxorubicin or epirubicin compared with cTACE,[10,14,15] and the rate of tumor progression at 12 months with the first anticancer drug was significantly lower in the DEB arm than in the bland embolization arm (46% vs 78%; $P \frac{1}{4} = .002$); TTP increased from 36.2 ± 9.0 weeks to 42.4 ± 9.5 weeks ($P \frac{1}{4} = .008$).[1,16] Moreover, epirubicin-loaded DEB versus cTACE shows a higher percentage of necrosis tumor observed in explanted livers (approximately 77% of lesions vs 27% with bland chemoembolization).[1,4]

Several TACE-related adverse events can occur in a significant proportion of patients, including ascites, depletion of liver function, infection (liver abscess), gastrointestinal bleeding, and postembolization syndrome comprising fever and abdominal pain.[5,6,17]

Despite these technological advances, the long-term survival of patients treated with TACE is unsatisfactory, mainly as a result of the high rates of tumor recurrence caused by progression of lesions not detected at the time of the procedure or the development of new lesions or loss of effectiveness of repeated doses of TACE (so-called TACE failure/refractoriness),[1,18] seen in scattered multifocal nodules in both lobes or a huge HCC mass, and the normal liver tissue deteriorates because of the damage caused by TACE, resulting in a reduced survival time. As a result, it has become apparent in recent years that the treatment modality should be switched before patients enter this state. This concept was first proposed by the Japan Society of Hepatology (JSH) and updated by the Liver Cancer Study Group of Japan (LCSGJ) in June 2014. Some specific features are considered to evaluate TACE failure/refractoriness, and these are listed in **Box 1**. An important point in this consensus is the need to subgroup intermediate-stage HCCs to improve response rate success.[18] The group of patients who would benefit from TACE comprises those with intermediate-stage HCC with 4 to 7 nodules of 3.4 cm in size, making long-term survival possible.

A median survival of 2 years (in almost 63% of patients) has been reported in a cohort of 104 Western patients with HCC treated with TACE compared with a control group (27%), but the effectiveness of this seems to depend on careful patient selection as mentioned earlier: compensated cirrhosis

---

Box 1
Definition of TACE failure/refractoriness

1. Intrahepatic lesion

   a. Two or more consecutive insufficient responses of the treated tumor (viable lesion >50%) even after changing the chemotherapeutic agents and/or reanalysis of the feeding artery seen on response evaluation CT/MR imaging at 1 to 3 months after having adequately performed selective TACE.

   b. Two or more consecutive progressions in the liver (tumor number increases compared with tumor number before the previous TACE procedure) even after having changed the chemotherapeutic agents and/or reanalysis of the feeding artery seen on response evaluation CT/MR imaging at 1 to 3 months after having adequately performed selective TACE.

2. Continuous increase of tumor markers immediately after TACE even though a slight transient decrease is observed

3. Appearance of vascular invasion

4. Appearance of extrahepatic spread

(Child-Pugh A), absence of cancer-related symptoms (Eastern Cooperative Oncology Group performance status of 0), and a large or multinodular HCC with neither vascular invasion nor extrahepatic spread.[1,19] However, there is a study (Cochrane meta-analysis) that shows contradictory evidence supporting that TACE does not have a beneficial effect on survival in patients with intermediate-grade HCC[20]; meanwhile some other experts have questioned this conclusion and expressed concern over this review.

In contrast, the high incidence of tumor recurrence in patients with HCC (22.3%, 65%, and 78% for the 6-month, 12-month, and 36-month cumulative rates, respectively) is explained to some extent by the increase in both plasma vascular endothelial growth factor (VEGF) levels and VEGF expression in the residual surviving cancerous hepatic tissue after TACE that leads to an upregulation in hypoxia-inducible factor 1-alpha, which in turn upregulates VEGF and increases tumor angiogenesis.[1,14,18,21] Thus, the combination of TACE, especially DEB-TACE, with antiangiogenic agents (sorafenib) is appealing because the systemically active drug (with activity on both tumor cells and endothelial cells) might curtail the post-TACE increase in VEGF-mediated signaling and at the same time target any tumor foci distant from the site of treatment.

The phase II randomized, double-blind, placebo-controlled SPACE (Sorafenib or Placebo in Combination with DEB-TACE for Intermediate-Stage HCC) study was the first global trial of the use of TACE in the treatment of HCC. Of 452 patients screened, 307 were randomized to sorafenib (n $1/4$ = 154) or placebo (n $1/4$ = 153), and the TTP for DEB-TACE plus sorafenib was longer than the TTP for DEB-TACE plus placebo.

However, Liu and colleagues[22] concluded in their meta-analysis that combination therapy with sorafenib and TACE may bring benefits for patients with unresectable HCC in terms of TTP but not overall survival (OS). Understanding the features of HCC and patient health that may predict the clinical outcome of combination regimens is therefore essential for prescribing individualized evidence-based therapeutic strategies.[4,23]

RADIOEMBOLIZATION

This technique involves the delivery of selective internal high-dose radiation via the hepatic artery. It represents an alternative form of therapy for BCLC-B HCC. This novel technique consists of the delivering of radioactive microspheres into the feeding arteries of the tumor so that the tumor nodules are treated irrespective of their location, number, or size.[4,24–26] The most important radioembolization technique currently uses microspheres coated with yttrium 90 (^{90}Y) beta-emitting isotope. Radioembolization has shown similar results to cTACE for survival, but longer TTP and less toxicity than cTACE. Salem and colleagues[27] showed that patients who received this treatment gained increased quality of life compared with patients who received cTACE.

PRETREATMENT IMAGING

Obtaining triple-phase computed tomography (CT) or MR imaging of the liver is mandatory to integrate clinical and laboratory data in the evaluation of the appropriateness of TACE by the local multidisciplinary liver tumor board. Additional imaging examinations to rule out extrahepatic disease should be performed as appropriate.

ASSESSMENT OF TREATMENT RESPONSE

Conventional methods for tumor response evaluation, such as Response Evaluation Criteria in Solid Tumors (RECIST), had no predictive value in patients with HCC who underwent cTACE or DEB-TACE because their criteria rely on tumor shrinkage as a measure of anticancer activity.[1,10,28,29]

Tumor response assessed by a modification of the RECIST criteria, named the modified RECIST (mRECIST), after TACE therapy for HCC is based on the fact that diameter of the targeted HCC tumors with viable tumor should guide all measurements and has been shown to correlate well with survival. Partial response (PR) is at least a 30% decrease in the sum of the diameters of viable (contrast enhancement in the arterial phase) lesions. Progressive disease (PD) is an increase of at least 20% in the sum of the diameters of viable lesions; stable disease denotes any cases that do not qualify as either PR or PD. Complete response (CR) is the disappearance of any intratumoral arterial enhancement in all lesions. OR included CR and PR.[30,31]

Furthermore, assessment of vascular invasion, lymph nodes, ascites, pleural effusion, and new lesions has been introduced. The EASL and the European Organization for Research and Treatment of Cancer (EORTC) have recently included in their clinical practice guidelines the use of the mRECIST for the assessment of treatment response in HCC therapy by performing multiphasic contrast-enhanced CT (CECT) or MR imaging 4 weeks after initial therapy for HCC.[4,10,32]

Multiphasic CECT is commonly used as a standard imaging technique for evaluating therapeutic response of TACE and performing surveillance of viable tumors in patients with HCC. However, radiologic imaging is not the best technique to determine tumor viability after TACE, because the retained hyperattenuating lipiodol material makes it difficult to detect contrast enhancement inside a viable tumor, giving only 43% accuracy.[30,33–37] MR imaging is better than CT, but the overall accuracy is less than 60%.

The most useful imaging modality to identify viable tumor versus tumor necrosis currently is PET scan, providing in vivo metabolic information with high sensitivity for detecting several primary and metastatic diseases.

Although ^{18}F-fluorodeoxyglucose (FDG) is the most widely used radiotracer for such studies, it has limited use in the diagnosis of primary HCCs because of the low expression of glucose transporter type 1 and the high levels of glycolytic enzymes, such as hexokinase type II (also known as glucose-6-phosphatase), especially in well-differentiated and low-grade HCCs, which dephosphorylate the intracellular glucose-6-phosphate delivering it back to the systemic circulation.[30,38–40]

In contrast, in large or high-grade HCCs, ^{18}F-FDG shows increased uptake correlating with high levels of serum alfa-fetoprotein (AFP) concentrations, indicating that AFP is involved in glucose metabolism and cell proliferation in pretreatment-naive HCC.[30,41] In summary, as mentioned before, ^{18}F-FDG-PET scans have poor sensitivity in the primary diagnosis of HCCs (50%–55%), which may be the reason why its diagnostic value in patients with HCCs treated with TACE is not widely known.

Chen and colleagues[42] reported that ^{18}F-FDG-PET detected 20 of 30 (67%) recurrent HCCs in patients showing increasing AFP concentrations after SR or interventional therapy, when results of conventional examinations were normal. These findings suggest that ^{18}F-FDG-PET/CT may be useful for detecting viable lipiodolized HCCs in patients with increased serum AFP but in whom no demonstrable viability is seen on multiphasic CECT images (Fig. 1).

There are some reports in the international literature that have examined the effectiveness of ^{18}F-FDG-PET or PET/CT in the assessment of tumor viability after TACE. However, not all studies included a wide range of patients; or they included patients with not only HCCs but hepatic metastasis tumors; not all of the subjects underwent TACE, PET, or PET/CT scans; and results were not always compared with CECT. These differences resulted in varying conclusions.[30,38,43–45]

The presence of residual viable tumor tissue was suggested by Torizuka and colleagues[44] as producing increased or similar ^{18}F-FDG uptake by a tumor with respect to surrounding normal tissue, whereas decreased or absent ^{18}F-FDG uptake indicated greater than 90% necrosis, showing that therapy had been effective.[30]

Kim and colleagues[30] performed an ^{18}F-FDG-PET/CT scan before and after treatment in 55 of 149 patients with HCC. None of these patients had small tumors (2 cm), diabetes, an interval from PET/CT to surgery longer than 1 month, invasive procedures between PET/CT and surgery, or systemic chemotherapy before or after PET/CT.

Multiphasic CECT images were obtained in all patients with a mean interval between this imaging and PET/CT of 4.1 to 14.3 days, considering lipiodolized HCC viable when the lesion showed arterial phase enhancement and defined tumor viability after TACE if the lipiodolized HCC score was grade II or grade III on both attenuation-corrected and non–attenuation-corrected PET images (grade I uptake was defined as no ^{18}F-FDG in the tumor or uptake that was less than in the surrounding normal liver; grade II was ^{18}F-FDG uptake similar to that in the surrounding normal liver; grade III was ^{18}F-FDG uptake greater than in the surrounding liver).

Tumor size was determined by histologic examination as the longest diameter, and differentiation was graded using the Edmonson-Steiner classification, with grades I and II defined as low and grades III and IV as high.[30,46]

The investigators analyzed ^{18}F-FDG uptake of the HCCs according the tumor size, pathologic grade, serum AFP concentration, presence of liver cirrhosis, and time interval between TACE and PET/CT. They identified 29 of the 30 viable lipiodolized HCCs (97%) with PET/CT and only 26 (86%) of them with multiphasic CECT. In 6 patients they had discordant results, with 3 true-positive viable HCCs seen by PET/CT and reported as false-negatives on CT. The other 3 nonviable HCCs were true-negatives on CECT.[30] PET findings more accurately reflected tumor viability than did intratumoral lipiodol retention on CT.

In addition, there was good correlation between grade and size of treatment-naive HCCs and the ^{18}F-FDG uptake, but not with AFP concentration, perhaps because increase of AFP level can also occur in benign disorders; 65% of low-grade and 62% of high-grade viable lipiodolized HCCs, compared with 37% of low-grade and 75% of

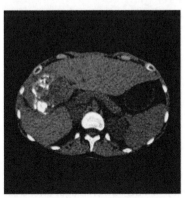 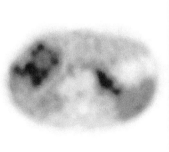 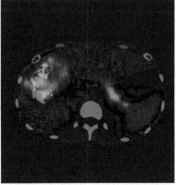

Fig. 1. Representative ^{18}F-FDG-PET/CT images of a 45-year-old woman with unresectable HCC after TACE. There is increased activity in the whole lesion compared with surrounding liver, consistent with persistent tumor viability.

high-grade treatment-naive HCCs, showed increased ^{18}F-FDG uptake (**Fig. 2**).

Note that similar results in ^{18}F-FDG uptake were obtained in lipiodolized HCCs independently of the tumor grade, in contrast with treatment-naive tumors, perhaps because the increased glycolysis in anaerobic conditions in residual tumors after TACE, as well as the hypoxia-inducible factor 1a protein expression in HCCs treated with TACE, tends to induce hexokinase II messenger RNA expression, mediating a phenotypic change and enabling cells to adapt to a hypoxic environment, allowing cancer cells to obtain sufficient energy for growth under the conditions of acute hypoxia or anoxia. One of these arrangements is the stimulation of angiogenesis through the overexpression of some synergistic growth (angiogenic) factors (vascular endothelial and basic fibroblast).[30]

An important cause of false-positives observed in ^{18}F-FDG uptake in the early postembolic period after TACE is the inflammatory reaction in the surrounding liver tissue with extravasation of inflammatory cells such as neutrophils, lymphocytes, and macrophages that accumulate ^{18}F-FDG in high proportions, contributing to the overall ^{18}F-FDG uptake in nonviable lipiodolized HCCs as well in viable tumors within approximately the first 3 months after TACE[47,48] (**Fig. 3**).

Another cause of false-positive results in PET/CT studies is respiratory motion artifacts and the undercorrection of attenuation caused by the presence of highly attenuating materials such as barium, metal, or lipiodol seen in the corrected images. It therefore becomes necessary to review the uncorrected images to help differentiate between artifacts and lesions, especially if the lesion is located in the periphery of the liver.[30]

In addition, the investigators considered that there is no absolute threshold for determining tumor viability, because standardized uptake value (SUV; the most commonly used quantitative measurement of ^{18}F-FDG uptake) can be influenced by many factors other than glucose metabolism.

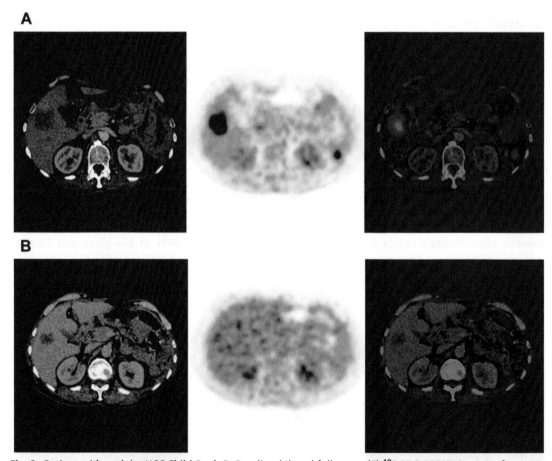

Fig. 2. Patient with nodular HCC Child-Pugh B. Baseline (*A*) and follow-up (*B*) ^{18}F-FDG-PET/CT images after treatment with TACE. (*A*) Note the abnormal increased uptake within the lesion. (*B*) After TACE there is an important reduction in size as well as metabolic activity in the lesion, suggesting complete metabolic response.

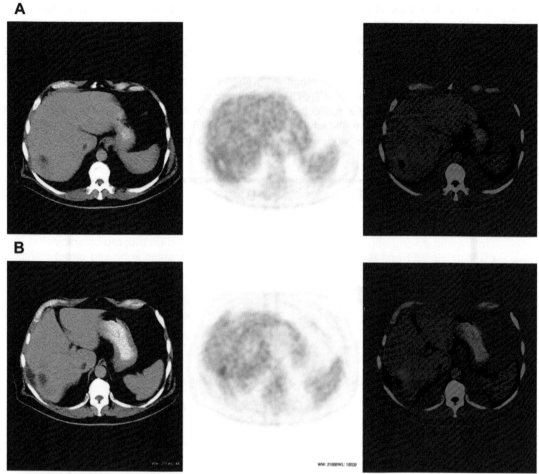

Fig. 3. ^{18}F-FDG-PET/CT transaxial images of an 65-year-old patient with HCC who underwent TACE. (*A*) Images were acquired 8 weeks after an interventionist procedure. Note the ring-shaped uptake of ^{18}F-FDG, suggesting inflammatory changes, but a focal abnormal increased ^{18}F-FDG uptake in the upper slices (*B*) that suggests residual tumor activity, which was confirmed by histopathology.

Nonetheless, the difference in ^{18}F-FDG uptake between a tumor and the liver can be expressed as an SUV ratio (T_{SUV}/L_{SUV}), which is associated with prognostic aspects of tumor aggressiveness such as differentiation grade, tumor size/number, and tumor recurrence in LT, therefore it is considered to have possible prognostic value in the treatment response in HCC.[31,49]

Song and colleagues,[31,45] in a retrospective study, showed the potential of ^{18}F-FDG uptake to predict treatment response for HCC with transarterial chemolipiodolization (TACL) with epirubicin or cisplatin (50 and 60 mg/m^2, respectively) followed by systemic chemoinfusion of 5-fluorouracil (200 mg/m^2).[50,51]

Treatment response was evaluated at 1 month after receiving 3 cycles of TACL by mRECIST. According to OR, patients with HCC were categorized into either an OR group or a nonresponse group. Some clinical features, including AFP, liver enzymes, and the $T_{suvmax}/L_{suvmean}$ ratio, were evaluated in both groups.

Because ^{18}F-FDG uptake is affected by underlying liver cirrhosis, the ratio more strongly reflects the underlying variation of glucose metabolism in the liver than the SUV of the tumor, so the SUV ratio in ^{18}F-FDG-PET diagnosis before treatment is an independent predictor of survival in unresectable patients with HCC because it correlates with tumor volume doubling time and the differentiation of HCC. The tumor/nontumor ratio of SUV may be an effective parameter of progression or aggressiveness in HCC.[31,52,53]

Furthermore, ^{18}F-FDG uptake between tumor (T_{suvmax}) and the normal liver ($L_{suvmean}$) showed the potential to predict treatment response with a cutoff $T_{suvmax}/L_{suvmean}$ value of 1.90. OR rates were significantly different at greater than

(77.7%) and less than (23.6%) the cutoff value (P<.001). In the univariate analysis, tumor size, portal vein thrombosis, and BCLC stage were significant as the $T_{suvmax}/L_{suvmean}$ ratio. However, in the multivariate analysis, $T_{suvmax}/L_{suvmean}$ was a significant prognostic factor with BCLC stage. This result suggests that the ratio of ^{18}F-FDG uptake might provide additional information (biological activity) to staging system, which has been used to predict outcome and inform decisions about treatment strategy in HCC[31,45,54] (Fig. 4).

Song and colleagues[35] also evaluated in a retrospective study the efficacy of ^{18}F-FDG-PET/CT in detecting viable tumor in 73 Asian patients with 91 HCCs after TACE and compared the diagnostic accuracy of ^{18}F-FDG-PET/CT with that of CECT. Furthermore, they assessed the value of ^{18}F-FDG-PET as a prognostic technique for the prediction of treatment response in HCC.

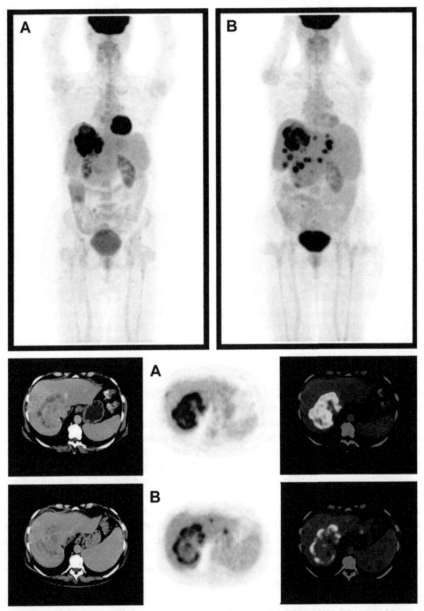

Fig. 4. ^{18}F-FDG-PET maximal intensity projection images and transaxial PET/CT of a 59-year-old woman with HCC after TACE treatment. (*A*) Extensive lesion covering almost the entire right lobe of the liver with high radiotracer uptake and slight deposition of lipiodol (<20%). Four-month follow-up PET/CT images (*B*) show PR in the primary lesion but intrahepatic spread, supporting progression of disease.

They used visual and semiquantitative criteria to describe the viability of HCC after TACE compared with the tracer uptake by normal liver parenchyma; in the visual judgment they used a 3-point grading system (hypometabolic, isometabolic, and hypermetabolic) and in the semiquantitative analysis they drew 1.5-cm regions of interest to calculate SUV_{max} in all lesions, and SUV_{mean} in normal liver, to subsequently evaluate $T_{suvmax}/L_{suvmean}$, considering a cutoff ratio of 1.65 to predict the response of HCC to TACE-based treatment. The SUV ratio of ^{18}F-FDG uptake was also an independent prognostic factor for OS in the multivariate analysis.

On a lesion-based analysis, among the 91 lesions of the 73 patients with HCC, the overall accuracy of ^{18}F-FDG-PET/CT was significantly higher than that of CECT (80.22% vs 67.03%; $P^{1/4} = .04$) for detecting viable tumor (52 hypermetabolic lesions), analyzing both attenuation-correction and non–attenuation-correction PET images. Inflammatory changes after TACE treatment must be considered to avoid false-positive results. Therefore, PET/CT should be performed 1 month after interventional treatment in order to reduce the incidence of false-positive results. The mean interval between the treatment of TACE and PET/CT was 41 days, with a range of 27 to 73 days.

Song and colleagues[35] suggested that ^{18}F-FDG uptake patterns of viable tumors can manifest as arc-shaped or punctate on the tumor periphery. This finding might be explained by the theory of dual blood supply (hepatic artery and portal vein) of HCC, considering that central blood supply is mainly from the hepatic artery and the peripheral blood supply from the portal vein. When hepatic artery is blocked by TACE, the peripheral tumor tends to form angiogenesis and the residual tumor survives, especially for lesions greater than 5 cm in diameter, which is why a large rimlike effect could suggest inflammation and a more eccentric focus is more likely to be caused by tumors. This finding indicates that tumor viability is assessed not only by whether there is ^{18}F-FDG uptake but also by the ^{18}F-FDG uptake pattern.

Song and colleagues[35] also analyzed the median survival times, concluding that the OS rate was significantly higher in the low-SUV-ratio group ($P^{1/4} = .024$) with a median of 40 months compared with 35 months in the high-SUV-ratio group.

For patients with HCC with a high SUV ratio, TACE alone may be insufficient to control tumor progression, and the addition of other treatment modalities early in the treatment period should be considered, such as radiofrequency ablation (RFA) and sorafenib.

In addition, Kim and colleagues[55] evaluated the prognostic value of ^{18}F-FDG uptake in 135 locally advanced HCCs that received localized concurrent chemoradiation therapy (a combination of intra-arterial chemotherapy and localized three-dimensional conformal radiation therapy).

Patients received external beam radiotherapy at 45 Gy for 5 weeks plus concurrent hepatic arterial infusion of 5-fluorouracil during the first and fifth week followed by repetitive hepatic arterial infusional chemotherapy with 5-fluorouracil and cisplatin, obtaining a considerable antitumor effect, with a median progression-free survival (PFS) of 6.5 months and an OS of 12.6 months, suggesting a benefit compared with the best supportive care and at least comparable outcomes compared with sorafenib in patients with locally advanced HCC. The SUV values calculated gave a median maximal SUV of 6.1. Patients with low maximal tumor SUVs (<6.1) had higher disease control rates than those with high maximal tumor SUVs (>6.1) and correlated with longer PFS and OS.

Therefore, ^{18}F-FDG-PET/CT has a high accuracy for detection of viable tumor in patients with HCC after TACE and may provide valuable information for prediction of treatment response; it could guide the optimal treatment (combined strategy) in those patients with HCCs with a high SUV ratio by providing a more aggressive locoregional therapy or a concomitant treatment rather than conventional TACE, in order to improve survival rates.[31,45,55]

REFERENCES

1. Lencioni R, Pasquale P, Crocetti L. Chemoembolization of hepatocellular carcinoma. Semin Intervent Radiol 2013;30:3–11.
2. Adhoute X, Penaranda G, Naude S, et al. Retreatment with TACE: the ABCR SCORE, an aid to the decision-making process. J Hepatol 2015;62(4): 855–62.
3. Tavernier J, Fagnoni P, Chabrot P, et al. Comparison of two transarterial chemoembolization strategies for hepatocellular carcinoma. Anticancer Res 2014;34: 7247–54.
4. Nishikawa H, Kita R, Kimura T, et al. Transcatheter arterial embolic therapies for hepatocellular carcinoma: a literature review. Anticancer Res 2014;34: 6877–86.
5. Lencioni R, Crocetti L. Local-regional treatment of hepatocellular carcinoma. Radiology 2012;262: 43–58.
6. Takayasu K. Transcatheter arterial chemoembolization for unresectable hepatocellular carcinoma: recent progression and perspective. Oncology 2013;84:28–33.

7. Doyon DMA, Jourde AM, Regensberg C, et al. L'embolisation arterielle hepatique dans les tumeurs malignes du foie. Ann Radiol 1974;17:593–603.

8. Yumoto Y, Jinno K, Tokuyama K, et al. Hepatocellular carcinoma detected by iodized oil. Radiology 1985; 154:19–24.

9. Ohishi H, Uchida H, Yoshimura H, et al. Hepatocellular carcinoma detected by iodized oil. Use of anti-cancer agents. Radiology 1985;154:25–9.

10. European Association for the Study of the Liver, European Organisation for Research and Treatment of Cancer. EASL-EORTC clinical practice guidelines: management of hepatocellular carcinoma. J Hepatol 2012;56:908–43.

11. Lencioni R. Loco-regional treatment of hepatocellular carcinoma. Hepatology 2010;52:762–73.

12. Varela M, Real MI, Burrel M, et al. Chemoembolization of hepato-cellular carcinoma with drug eluting beads: efficacy and doxorubicin pharmacokinetics. J Hepatol 2007;46:474–81.

13. Lencioni R, de Baere T, Burrel M, et al. Transcatheter treatment of hepatocellular carcinoma with doxorubicin-loaded DC bead (DEB-DOX): technical recommendations. Cardiovasc Intervent Radiol 2012;35:980–5.

14. Lammer J, Malagari K, Vogl T, et al, PRECISION V Investigators. Prospective randomized study of doxorubicin-eluting-bead embolization in the treatment of hepatocellular carcinoma: results of the PRECISION V study. Cardiovasc Intervent Radiol 2010;33:41–52.

15. Kishimoto S, Noguchi T, Yamaoka T, et al. Antitumor effects of a novel lipophilic platinum complex (SM-11355) against a slowly growing rat hepatic tumor after intra-hepatic arterial administration. Biol Pharm Bull 2000;23:344–8.

16. Malagari K, Pomoni M, Kelekis A, et al. Prospective randomized comparison of chemoembolization with doxorubicin-eluting beads and bland embolization with BeadBlock for hepatocellular carcinoma. Cardiovasc Intervent Radiol 2010;33:541–51.

17. Miyayama S, Yamashiro M, Okuda M, et al. Usefulness of cone-beam computed tomography during ultraselective transcatheter arterial chemoembolization for small hepatocellular carcinomas that cannot be demonstrated on angiography. Cardiovasc Intervent Radiol 2009;32:255–64.

18. Kudoa M, Matsuib O, Izumic N, et al. Transarterial chemoembolization failure/refractoriness: JSH-LCSGJ criteria 2014 update. Oncology 2014;87: 22–31.

19. Burrel M, Reig M, Forner A, et al. Survival of patients with hepatocellular carcinoma treated by transarterial chemoembolisation (TACE) using drug eluting beads. Implications for clinical practice and trial design. J Hepatol 2012;56:1330–5.

20. Oliveri RS, Wetterslev J, Gluud C. Transarterial (chemo) embolisation for unresectable hepatocellular carcinoma. Cochrane Database Syst Rev 2011;(3):CD004787.

21. Lencioni R. Management of hepatocellular carcinoma with trans-arterial chemoembolization in the era of systemic targeted therapy. Crit Rev Oncol Hematol 2012;83:216–24.

22. Liu L, Chen H, Wang M, et al. Combination therapy of sorafenib and TACE for unresectable HCC: a systematic review and meta-analysis. PLoS One 2014; 9(3):e91124.

23. Hsu CY, Hsia CY, Huang YH, et al. Comparison of surgical resection and transarterial chemoembolization for hepatocellular carcinoma beyond the Milan criteria: a propensity score analysis. Ann Surg Oncol 2012;19(3):842–9.

24. Lau WY, Sangro B, Chen PJ, et al. Treatment for hepatocellular carcinoma with portal vein tumor thrombosis: the emerging role for radioembolization using yttrium-90. Oncology 2013;84:311–8.

25. Sangro B, Carpanese L, Cianni R, et al. Survival after yttrium-90 resin microsphere radioembolization of hepatocellular carcinoma across Barcelona clinic liver cancer stages: a European evaluation. Hepatology 2011;54:868–78.

26. Golfieri R, Bilbao JI, Carpanese L, et al. Comparison of the survival and tolerability of radioembolization in elderly vs. younger patients with unresectable hepatocellular carcinoma. J Hepatol 2013;59:753–61.

27. Salem R, Gilbertsen M, Butt Z, et al. Increased quality of life among hepatocellular carcinoma patients treated with radioembolization, compared with chemoembolization. Clin Gastroenterol Hepatol 2013; 11:1358–65.

28. Forner A, Ayuso C, Varela M, et al. Evaluation of tumor response after locoregional therapies in hepatocellular carcinoma: are response evaluation criteria in solid tumors reliable? Cancer 2009;30:616–23.

29. Bruix J, Sherman M. Management of hepatocellular carcinoma: an update. Hepatology 2011;53:1020–2.

30. Kim HO, Kim JS, Shin YM, et al. Evaluation of metabolic characteristics and viability of lipiodolized hepatocellular carcinomas using 18F-FDG PET/CT. J Nucl Med 2010;51:1849–56.

31. Song MJ, Bae SH, Yoo IeR, et al. Predictive value of 18F-fluorodeoxyglucose PET/CT for transarterial chemolipiodolization of hepatocellular carcinoma. World J Gastroenterol 2012;18:3215–22.

32. Lencioni R, Llovet J. M: modified RECIST (mRECIST) assessment for hepatocellular carcinoma. Semin Liver Dis 2010;30:52–60.

33. Takayasu K, Arii S, Matsuo N, et al. Comparison of CT findings with resected specimens after chemoembolization with iodized oil for hepatocellular carcinoma. AJR Am J Roentgenol 2000;175:699–704.

34. Guan YS, Sun L, Zhou XP, et al. Hepatocellular carcinoma treated with interventional procedures: CT and MRI follow-up. World J Gastroenterol 2004;10: 3543–8.

35. Song HJ, Cheng JY, Hu SL, et al. Value of 18F-FDG PET/CT in detecting viable tumour and predicting prognosis of hepatocellular carcinoma after TACE. Clin Radiol 2014;70(2):128–37.

36. Brown DB, Nikolic B, Covey AM, et al. Quality improvement guidelines for transhepatic arterial chemoembolization, embolization, and chemotherapeutic infusion for hepatic malignancy. J Vasc Interv Radiol 2012;23:287–94.

37. Hunt SJ, Yu W, Weintraub J, et al. Radiologic monitoring of hepatocellular carcinoma tumor viability after transhepatic arterial chemo-embolization: estimating the accuracy of contrast-enhanced cross-sectional imaging with histopathologic correlation. J Vasc Interv Radiol 2009;20:30–8.

38. Okazumi S, Isono K, Enomoto K, et al. Evaluation of liver tumors using fluorine-18-fluorodeoxyglucose PET: characterization of tumor and assessment of effect of treatment. J Nucl Med 1992;33:333–9.

39. Torizuka T, Tamaki N, Inokuma T, et al. In vivo assessment of glucose metabolism in hepatocellular carcinoma with FDG-PET. J Nucl Med 1995;36: 1811–7.

40. Iwata Y, Shiomi S, Sasaki N, et al. Clinical usefulness of positron emission tomography with fluorine-18-fluorodeoxyglucose in the diagnosis of liver tumors. Ann Nucl Med 2000;14:121–6.

41. Shang JB, Li YH, Liu FY, et al. 18F-Fluorodeoxyglucose uptake in hepatocellular carcinoma on positron emission tomography correlates with alpha-fetoprotein. Di Yi Jun Yi Da Xue Xue Bao 2004;24:697–9.

42. Chen YK, Hsieh DS, Liao CS, et al. Utility of FDG-PET for investigating unexplained serum AFP elevation in patients with suspected hepatocellular carcinoma recurrence. Anticancer Res 2005;25: 4719–25.

43. Vitola JV, Delbeke D, Meranze SG, et al. Positron emission tomography with F-18-fluorodeoxyglucose to evaluate the results of hepatic chemoembolization. Cancer 1996;78:2216–22.

44. Torizuka T, Tamaki N, Inokuma T, et al. Value of fluorine-18-FDG-PET to monitor hepatocellular carcinoma after interventional therapy. J Nucl Med 1994;35:1965–9.

45. Song MJ, Bae SH, Lee SW, et al. (18)F-Fluorodeoxyglucose PET/CT predicts tumour progression after transarterial chemoembolization in hepatocellular carcinoma. Eur J Nucl Med Mol Imaging 2013;40: 865–73.

46. Edmondson HA, Steiner PE. Primary carcinoma of the liver: a study of 100 cases among 48,900 necropsies. Cancer 1954;7:462–503.

47. Jiang B, Lou Q, Ding XF, et al. Histopathological changes in rat transplanted hepatoma after lipiodol transarterial embolization. Zhonghua Zhong Liu Za Zhi 2004;26:205–8.

48. Meller J, Sahlmann C-O, Scheel AK. 18F-FDG PET and PET/CT in fever of unknown origin. J Nucl Med 2007;48:35–45.

49. Yang SH, Suh KS, Lee HW, et al. The role of (18) F-FDG-PET imaging for the selection of liver transplantation candidates among hepatocellular carcinoma patients. Liver Transpl 2006;12:1655–60.

50. Kirchhoff TD, Rudolph KL, Layer G, et al. Chemoocclusion vs chemoperfusion for treatment of advanced hepatocellular carcinoma: a randomised trial. Eur J Surg Oncol 2006;32:201–7.

51. Jang JW, Bae SH, Choi JY, et al. A combination therapy with transarterial chemolipiodolization and systemic chemo-infusion for large extensive hepatocellular carcinoma invading portal vein in comparison with conservative management. Cancer Chemother Pharmacol 2007;59:9–15.

52. Megyesi C, Samols E, Marks V. Glucose tolerance and diabetes in chronic liver disease. Lancet 1967; 2:1051–6.

53. Petrides AS, DeFronzo RA. Glucose metabolism in cirrhosis: a review with some perspectives for the future. Diabetes Metab Rev 1989;5:691–709.

54. Llovet JM, Brú C, Bruix J. Prognosis of hepatocellular carcinoma: the BCLC staging classification. Semin Liver Dis 1999;19:329–38.

55. Kim BK, Kang WJ, Kim JK, et al. 18F-Fluorodeoxyglucose uptake on positron emission tomography as a prognostic predictor in locally advanced hepatocellular carcinoma. Cancer 2011;117:4779–87.

PET/Computed Tomography and Thermoablation (Radiofrequency, Microwave, Cryotherapy, Laser Interstitial Thermal Therapy)

Françoise Bonichon, MD, MSc[a],*, Yann Godbert, MD[a],
Afshin Gangi, MD, PhD[b], Xavier Buy, MD[c],
Jean Palussière, MD[c]

KEYWORDS

- Thermal ablation • Radiofrequency • Microwave • Cryosurgery • Laser interstitial thermal therapy
- PET/CT • FDG • Local control

KEY POINTS

- Thermal ablation is increasingly used in oncology for primary and secondary cancer but is also used to destroy benign tumors.
- PET/computed tomography (CT) plays an important role in the follow-up to detect residual viable tissue and early detection of a relapse that can be re-treated by thermal ablation or other means.
- Postablation aspects have to be well known by the specialist in charge of image interpretation.
- All studies are concordant to conclude that PET/CT is a useful tool for early recognition of incomplete tumor destruction after thermal ablation.

INTRODUCTION

Image-guided thermal ablation is an evolving and growing treatment option for patients with malignant disease of multiple organ systems. Treatment indications have been expanded to include benign tumors as well. Specifically, the most prevalent indications to date have been in the liver (primary and metastatic disease), the lungs (metastatic disease or primary lung cancer), kidney (primarily renal cell carcinoma, but also benign tumors such as angiomyolipomas and oncocytomas), and soft tissue and bone (metastatic disease and osteoid osteomas or osteoblastoma). In the past, for the same indications, the treatment of choice was surgery, but thermal ablation is safe, feasible in patients who have surgical contraindications, and easily repeatable. The goal of this article is to perform a literature review on the role of PET/computed tomography (CT) in thermal ablation, its indications, accuracy, timing, and limits in different indications. The authors performed a PubMed search from the beginning until December 31, 2014 using a Mijnhout-adapted search strategy[1,2] combined with the following

The authors have nothing to disclose.
[a] Department of Nuclear Medicine, Institut Bergonié, 229 cours de l'Argonne, Bordeaux 33000, France; [b] Non-Vascular IR Department, University Hospital of Strasbourg, Nouvel hopital civil, 1 Place de l'hopital, BP 426, Strasbourg 67091, France; [c] Department of Interventional Radiology, Institut Bergonié, 229 cours de l'Argonne, Bordeaux 33000, France
* Corresponding author.
E-mail address: f.bonichon@bordeaux.unicancer.fr

PET Clin 10 (2015) 519–540
http://dx.doi.org/10.1016/j.cpet.2015.05.008

PubMed terms: ablation techniques [MESH], cryosurgery [MESH], cryotherapy [all fields], radiofrequency [all fields], microwave [all fields], "thermal ablation" [all fields], laser ablation [MESH], "Laser induced thermal ablation" [all fields], lasers/therapeutic use [MESH]. For lung or liver tumors, case reports were excluded. For the other lesions, small series as well as case reports were included.

DIFFERENT THERMOABLATION TECHNIQUES

The goal of thermal ablation is to destroy the involved tissue by heating (radiofrequency, microwaves, laser) or by freezing (cryotherapy).

All these techniques are percutaneous or intraoperative (for some liver metastases) and require biologic workup, including coagulation, and an anesthesia visit, although some thermal ablations may be performed under local anesthesia or sedation. The opinion of an interventional radiologist as to technical feasibility should always be sought, and indication must be confirmed by a multidisciplinary team.

They also require strictly aseptic conditions and, if possible, intraoperative CT navigation.

Radiofrequency

Radiofrequency ablation (RFA) is a thermoablation technique in which a thin percutaneous (or intraoperative) electrode is introduced into or near the tumor and dispersion plates are positioned on the patient, creating an electric circuit with an alternating current from a 460- to 480-Hz radiofrequency generator. The current induces ionic agitation, heating the tumor and the surrounding area, destroying cells by protein denaturation and coagulative necrosis. It can be used for lung,[3] liver, bone metastases,[4] or primary lung, liver, kidney, or breast cancer, but also for some benign tumors (kidney angiomyolipoma or oncocytoma).

Radiofrequency is used in different domains, mainly in tumor destruction but also for reducing supraventricular tachyarrythmia[5] or ventricular tachycardia. This work was limited to PET/CT for tumor destruction by thermal ablation evaluation because only 3 papers were found describing integration of PET/CT with electroanatomical mapping for ablation of scar-related ventricular tachycardia,[6–8] and one paper was found describing sustained monomorphic ventricular tachycardia with mediastinal adenopathy.[9]

Microwave

Microwave-like RFA uses electromagnetic current, but in a frequency band of 900 to 2450 MHz.[10] Heating is faster and stronger than with radiofrequency, based on micromovement of water molecules. The theoretical advantages, which remain to be proven, are the possibility of treating lesions larger than 3 cm and avoiding heat loss around large vessels. Microwave ablation is a growing field with ongoing and published studies about its clinical utility, limitations, and safety.

Cryotherapy

Cryotherapy is a form of cold thermoablation. A probe is introduced into the tumor percutaneously. Freezing is achieved by circulation under pressure of a rare gas, argon, and rapid decompression induces cooling down to $-140°C$ by the Joule-Thomson effect. Less than $-20°C$, cell membranes are destroyed and proteins are denatured, causing cell death.[11] To maximize destruction, several freeze-thaw cycles are needed, with helium circulation to induce thawing. One session lasts about 30 minutes and does not necessarily require general anesthesia. The advantage of cryotherapy is that the iceball is visible on the CT, so that the treated volume can be estimated with precision. Similarly like other percutaneous techniques, hospital stay is short. Large volumes can be treated by parallel probes at intervals of about 2 cm. The drawback is the high cost of the needles and the rare gas. The theoretic risk of neural lesion around the treatment area can be avoided by precise temperature control or by using carbon dioxide or physiologic saline to push the protected structure out of the way.[12]

Laser Ablation

Laser ablation, also termed laser interstitial thermal therapy (LITT), uses optical fibers to transmit infrared light energy into a tumor to produce heat and coagulation necrosis.

GOALS OF THE PET/COMPUTED TOMOGRAPHY
Before the Thermal Ablation

- If the global workup for malignancies confirms there are not too many metastases (usually less than <5, thermal ablation is a good option). It is also important to check if the lesion is fluorodeoxyglucose (FDG)-avid. If not, PET/CT will be unusable after thermal ablation to detect a local recurrence.

During Thermal Ablation

PET/CT can guide the operator to put the needle or the probe in the most aggressive part of the lesion. This technique has been used in recent studies but is not a standard of care.

After Thermal Ablation

- Thermal ablation complications must be detected.
- It must be determined if there is a residual active lesion permitting early re-treatment and then improved survival.
- Other recurrences, nodal or distant, must be detected.

INTERPRETATION AND IMAGE PATTERNS

Using thermal ablation, the posttreatment images are the same whatever is the site of the metastase or the primary tumor, and these posttreatment aspects and their kinetics must be known and understood because these aspects are different from other posttreatment aspects, for example, after chemotherapy.

It is important to interpret not only the metabolic images and their changes but also the CT, which is part of the PET/CT.

Recognizing the normal FDG-PET appearances after thermal ablation is important to prevent misdiagnosis of local tumor progression (LTP).

Some animal models have helped the understanding of the posttreatment CT and PET images.[13–18]

RESULTS IN DIFFERENT SITUATIONS
Lung Malignancies

Minimally invasive techniques, such as RFA and radiowaves (MW), have been developed for the treatment of unresectable primary and secondary lung tumors mostly for patients with comorbidities that contraindicate surgery. The complications are frequent but often of low grade: transient pneumothorax (with or without drainage <48 hours) is the more frequent complication (40%).[19] The other complications are pleural effusion (19%), alveolar hemorrhage (5.9%), or rare complications, such as cavitation, lung abscess, pulmonary aspergilloma,[20] injury to the nearby tissues (nerves, ribs), systemic air embolism, needle track seeding, and skin burn.[21]

The repeatability and low morbidity of these techniques are great advantages. Treatment can be on an outpatient basis or with a short (less than 2 days) hospital stay.

The limitations of radiofrequency are

- Metastasis size, with much poorer efficacy beyond 3 cm;
- Proximity of large vessels, leading to heat loss and reduced efficacy (heat-sink effect);
- Proximity of the parietal pleura, which may lead to persistent pain; this can be prevented by creating a pneumothorax, and by holding the parietal pleura back during the procedure.

The nuclear medicine practitioner needs to be familiar with the posttreatment CT aspect in the lung[22] so as to not mistakenly suspect recurrence: the image after thermal ablation is always larger than the baseline image, and the Response Evaluation Criteria In Solid Tumors (RECIST)[23] criteria are not applicable.

Cryotherapy has been described as a salvage treatment after local relapse for an unresectable primary lung cancer, and it is not yet a standard option.[24]

Table 1 shows the studies using PET/CT for workup, prognosis, and local relapse evaluation of thermal ablation in lung malignancies. There are very few large prospective studies to evaluate accuracy of the PET/CT in this context. Furthermore, many studies mix primary and secondary lung malignancies, which do not have the same outcome.

Lung metastases

They were the first indications of thermal ablation specially when patients were at high risk of morbidity secondary to a potential thoracotomy or when patients refused surgery. In prospective trials there was low morbidity[25,26] and long survival was observed in selected patients with lung metastases from colorectal carcinoma[27] or soft tissue sarcoma.[28,29]

Non-small cell lung cancer

Primary lung cancer is the leading cause of cancer-related death worldwide. The suggested first-line treatment of early (T1N0M0) stage non-small cell lung cancer (NSCLC) is lobectomy, but more than 20% of cases are not good surgical candidates because of frequent comorbidities. These cases are usually treated by conventional external beam radiation therapy or more recently by stereotactic body radiotherapy (SBRT). RFA has been offered as an alternative treatment option for early-stage NSCLC for well over a decade with promising mid- to long-term results in tumors smaller than 3 cm. Radiofrequency or microwaves are useful options because of the low morbidity and short hospitalization stay. After radiofrequency, the 1-year overall survival is 78% to 95%.[30–33] A comparison of prospective studies shows an equivalence of local recurrence rates at 1 year.[34] After local recurrence, whatever was the first-line treatment radiofrequency can be a salvage treatment and can be applied even in irradiated zones.[35] Microwaves are always under evaluation in this indication but seem to be useful for older patients.[36] After thermal ablation, the local recurrence rate is greater than for thermal ablation of metastases, probably because of greater microscopic extension around the lesion.

Table 1
PET/computed tomography and different lung lesions

Author (Ref), Year	R/P	No. of Pts./Lesions	Technique	Type of Lung Cancer	Local Control	Timing of PET/CT	Remarks
Kang et al,[84] 2004	P	50/120	RFA	23 primary 27 M+	70%	1–2 wk	35 PET
Hataji et al,[85] 2005	R	11	RFA	7 recurrent primary 4 M+	Few if >3.5 cm	1 to 2 wk	Early PET unable to detect LTP. Cells persist at the periphery of the lesions (1 autopsy)
Okuma et al,[86] 2006	R	12/17	RFA	5 primary 7 M+	5 negative PET: no relapse 12 positive PET: 11 progressive disease	2 mo	PET visual analysis: Se, 100%; Sp: 83.3%, accuracy: 94.1%
Higaki et al,[87] 2008	R	15/60	RFA	4 primary 11 M+	10/60 LTP	1–9 mo	SUVmax = 1.5 Se = 77.8%, Sp = 90%
Lanuti et al,[31] 2009	R	31/31	RFA	Stage 1 inoperable NSCLC	68.5% no local relapse	≥3 mo	Local control = no eccentric FDG uptake on PET/CT at a minimum of 3 mo. Median survival 30 mo
Singnurkar et al,[43] 2010	R	68/94	RFA	44 primary 38 lesions M+	9/28 recurrences if favorable pattern 10/12 recurrences if unfavorable pattern	—	Description of image patterns, recurrences of primary cancer > metastases. PET progression can be preceded by 6 mo CT progression
Deandreis et al,[41] 2011	P	34/46	RFA	29 M+ 5 primary	4/46 (14%) incomplete treatment (14%) at 3 mo	24 h, 1 mo, 3 mo	PET+: focal uptake heterogeneous, SUVmax >2.5 1 false positive SUVmax = 7.1
Harada et al,[88] 2011	R	39	RFA	10 primary 29 M+	9/39 recurrences	Before RFA 1,3,6,9 then every 6 mo	Preablation SUVmax useful to predict local relapse

Study	Type	N	Treatment	Population	Local control / outcome	Follow-up timing	Comments
Yoo et al,[89] 2011	P	30	RFA	Stage 1 inoperable NSCLC	100% if 6 mo PET/CT negative	4 D, 1 and 6 mo	Early PET/CT at 4 d not useful; PET/CT at 6 mo useful
Lanuti et al,[35] 2012	R	—	—	Stage 1 inoperable NSCLC	100% with SBRT; 40% with repeated RFA	3 and 6 mo	Management of local recurrence after RFA
Schoellnast et al,[90] 2012	R	33	RFA	Recurrent primary NSCLC	Median TTLP: 24 mo if < 3 cm; 8 mo if ≥3 cm	Before RFA and after RFA if relapse suspicion	RFA useful as salvage therapy for NSCLC
Alafate et al,[91] 2013	R	25/30	RFA	9 primary, 16 M+	11 progression 3 mo; 15 stable 3 mo	3 and 6 mo	RECIST response evaluation on CT SUVmax after ARF
Bonichon et al,[40] 2013	P	89/115	RFA	M+ only	84.6% free of local recurrence at 1 y	1 and 3 mo	3 mo optimal different patterns
Gadaleta et al,[92] 2013	P	17/20	Chemoembolization + RFA	3 primary 17 lesions M+	100% if nodule <3 cm; 79% if nodule 3–5 cm	At 3 mo, then at every 6 mo	—
Kodama et al,[93] 2013	P	84	RFA	Colorectal cancer lung metastases	—	Before RFA	Importance of pre-RFA PET/CT to confirm RFA indication
Sharma et al,[94] 2013	R	18/19	RFA	14 Primary NSCLC/ 5 M+ without any progression after RFA	—	1, 3, 6, 12 mo	Increase of FDG uptake after complete RFA is not always a local relapse
Acksteiner & Steinke,[36] 2015	R	10/11	MWA	Primary NSCLC	3/11 LTP	At 3 or 12 mo if possible	MWA in elderly people (>75 y), avid FDG rim can persist until 6 mo because of inflammation
Higuchi et al,[95] 2014	P	20/24	RFA	6 primary 14 M+	2-y local control rate 74.3%	7–14 d, 3–6 mo	7–14 d SUVmax not correlated to recurrence; 3–6 mo SUVmax significantly correlated to recurrence

Abbreviations: M+, metastatic patient; MWA, microwaves; NA, not available; NPV, negative predictive value; P, prospective; R, retrospective; Se, sensitivity; Sp, specificity; SUV, standard uptake value; TTLP, time to local progression.

Images

No matter which technique is used, radiofrequency or microwaves, the postablated image is always larger than the preablated image because the surrounding normal tissues are also ablated as a safety margin to ensure complete ablation. Giraud and colleagues[37] studied the degree of local microscopic extension in primary lung cancer and have shown that a margin of 8 mm for adenocarcinoma and 6 mm for squamous cell carcinoma must be included in the conformal radiotherapy planning to be certain to cover 95% of microscopic extension. The goal of ablation should be to include an expected ablation zone that includes the primary tumor plus at least an additional 8–10 mm of ablation beyond the visible tumor margin in all directions as recommended by Beland and colleagues[38] for the treatment of primary lung tumor.

Computed Tomographic Scan

Usually CT imaging is performed 2 days after treatment and then at 2, 4, 6, 9, and 12 months. The goal of the 1 or 2 days of CT is to detect complications: pneumothorax, pleural effusion hemorrhage, lung abscess, and others.

On the early postablation CT, there is usually a ground-glass aspect of the margins around the nodule.

The goals of the subsequent CTs are to observe resolution of complications and to detect early local relapse to re-treat.

Different postablation images are well described in a prospective study by Palussiere and colleagues.[22] The different aspects are as follows:

- Atelectasis: Ventilatory disturbance in a segment with increased attenuation surrounding the ablated tumor, thus preventing analysis of the RFA ablated tumor.
- Cavitation: An air-filled cavity with thick or thin walls appearing in the location of the ablated area. Cavitation may be incomplete and only in one part of the ablated volume.
- Disappearance: The RFA zone is impossible to depict. No sequelae of the ablation zone are seen.
- Fibrosis: The RFA zone loses its sphericity and becomes elongated and linear with or without peripheral spicules.
- Nodule

LTP will be suspected after ablation if there is an increased size of the ablated zone on 2 subsequent CT follow-ups or if there is an appearance of an enhanced nodular focus on a contrast-enhanced CT (CECT).

PET/Computed Tomography

Different PET/CT image patterns are observed, and there is no consensus on what is normal postablation change and what is suspect of incomplete ablation of relapse.[39–43]

A normal postablation change has characteristics as follows:

- Nodular photopenic zone larger than the pre-ablation nodule (**Fig. 1**)
- Regular rim with faint FDG uptake around a photopenic zone (**Fig. 2**)

What is considered an incomplete ablation or local relapse:

- Irregular nodule at the periphery of ablated zone with intense FDG uptake

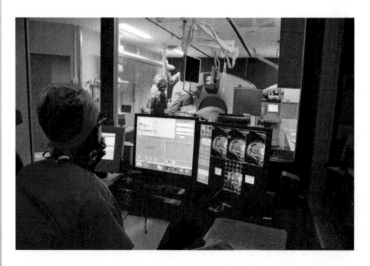

Fig. 1. RFA or cryotherapy CT guidance. On the CT screens, there is a grid that helps to introduce the electrode to the probe percutaneously into or near the target lesion (*arrows*).

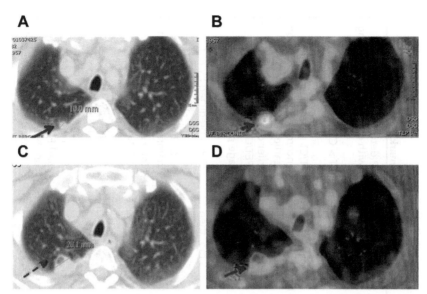

A

B

C

D

Fig. 2. True-negative PET/CT after RFA for lung metastasis. A 51-year-old man with papillary thyroid carcinoma pT4N1aM1, 2 years before. Unique lung metastases, with biopsy proven. Surgery contraindicated. (*A, B*) PET/CT before RFA (*red arrows*): 10-mm nodule with intense FDG uptake. (*C, D*) PET/CT 3 months after RFA (*red dashed arrows*). On CT (*C*), the image of the ablated zone is larger (20 mm) than preablated image (*red dashed arrow*). On the PET image (*D*), there is a central photopenic zone with a rim with faint FDG uptake near the pleura (*red arrow*). This image was considered negative, and the patient remains in complete clinical and biological remission 6 years later.

Timing of PET/Computed Tomography

It seems the best time to perform PET/CT follow-up is between 3 and 6 months to evaluate local response and to confirm local complete ablation.

Liver Malignancies

Local ablative therapies, especially thermal ablations, are being increasingly used for the purpose of providing local control of primary or secondary liver tumors while sparing normal liver tissue. RFA is the most often used, and cryotherapy[44] and microwave coagulation[45] are not yet standard of care for liver tumors.

Table 2 shows the studies using PET/CT for workup before RFA, prognosis, and local relapse evaluation of thermal ablation in liver malignancies.

Liver Metastases

Up to 25% of patients with cancer will develop metastases during the course of their disease, and this will cause morbidity and mortality. Colorectal cancer is the most common malignancy, leading to liver metastases, one of the most common malignant diseases in the world. In two-thirds of patients, colorectal liver metastases (CLM) are limited to liver, but few patients are good candidates for surgery because of morbidity, location of the lesion, the multifocality of metastases, an

impaired liver function, or metastases outside of the liver. Often chemotherapy is used, but some metastases are refractory to chemotherapy or there are toxicities that limit the use of chemotherapy. Sometimes there is good response to chemotherapy and if it remains only few liver metastases a local treatment is considered by the multidisciplinary team. In these cases, thermal ablation may be useful to obtain complete eradication of the metastases. The vast majority of studies concerns radiofrequency. The use of this technique for the treatment of CLM has been approved by the US Food and Drug Administration for several years, and this therapy is now being adopted worldwide. However, the risk of relapse after RFA is high (3.6%–60%), as shown by Wong and colleagues[46] in an evidence review of RFA of hepatic metastases from colorectal cancer. The results depend on location, multifocality, and size of metastases. Survival after RFA for CLM is good, equivalent to surgery for solitary CLM,[47] and better than with chemotherapy alone if the lesions are less than 3 cm.[48] It is challenging to find early the absence of residual disease. Usually this is done by CT or MRI and also by observation of decreasing biomarkers as carcinoembryonic antigen plasmatic level. Many studies shown in **Table 1** have evaluated the added value of PET/CT for the detection of LTP. All studies are concordant that PET/CT can find LTP earlier than CT or MRI. There is no consensus

Table 2
PET/computed tomography and thermal ablation of different liver lesions

Author (Ref), Year	R/P/M	No. of Pts./Lesions	Technique	Cancer Type	Local Control	Timing of PET/CT	Remarks
Langenhoff et al,[96] 2002	P	23/56	CRY/RFA	M+ CLM	5 FDG + in follow-up 4/5 developed local relapse	3, 6 wk, then every 3 mo	LTP detection earlier than with conventional imaging
Anderson et al,[97] 2003	R	13	RFA	M+	—	9 mo ± 5 mo	PET > CT; PET > MRI
Donckier et al,[98] 2003	R	17/28	RFA	M+	24/28 no residual tumor 13 relapses (4 FDG + CT−)	1 wk, 1 mo	PET/CT recognizes incomplete tumor ablation earlier than CT
Blokhuis et al,[99] 2004	R	15	RFA	1 Primary 14 M+	4 LTP at a mean of 9 mo	Various intervals in 11 pts	Earlier detection of LTP by PET/CT than CECT alone
Barker et al,[100] 2005	R	—	RFA	M+	—	W to mo	Image patterns after RFA
Joosten et al,[101] 2005	R	On early PR58	30 CRY ± resection, 28 RFA ± resection	M+	91% after CRY, 94% after RFA	3, 6 mo, then every 6 mo	7 LTP; 6 predicted by PET, none by CT
Amthauer et al,[102] 2006	R	68	LITT	M+ CLM	—	—	PET/CT before LITT to determine lesions to treat
Denecke et al,[103] 2007	R	21/54	LITT Clinical suspicion of tumor progression after LITT	M+ CLM	—	—	Faintly enhanced rim of increase activity interpreted as reactive changes SUVmax
Khandani et al,[104] 2007	P	8/8	RFA	M+	88% no inflammatory uptake at the early PET/CT 86% results predicted on early PET/CT	2–41 h after RFA	5 total photopenia on early PET/CT, 1 round focus at 8 mo with increasing size and FDG uptake intensity on the following PET/CT 2 intense uptake on the early PET/CT 1 rim-shaped uptake on the early PET/CT; 7 mo later focal uptake at the edge of the rim

Study							
Paudyal et al,[50] 2007	R	24/33	RFA	Primary HCC	50%	Pre-RFA 3, 6, 9, 12 mo, then every 6 mo	On the pre-RFA PET/CT only 50% FDG uptake. SUV max correlated to AFP level. PET/CT detected recurrence in 12 pts. Inverse correlation between initial SUV and time to recurrence PET/CT detects earlier and better recurrence than CT 2 detection of extrahepatic metastases
Kuehl et al,[105] 2008	P	16/25	RFA	CLM	12/25 lesions: LTP	24 h, 1, 3, 9 mo, then every 6 mo	PET/CT Se: 91%, accuracy: 83% better than PET, CT, MRI
Travaini et al,[106] 2008	R	9/12	RFA	M+	1 residual disease, 7 relapses/12 lesions	1 wk, 1, 3, 6, 9 mo	LTP detected earlier with PET/CT
Dierckx et al,[107] 2009	Revue	—	—	Primary, M+	—	—	—
Han et al,[108] 2009	R	18	RFA	Primary	—	—	Usefulness of PET/CT when unexplained increasing AFP after RFA or transarterial chemoembolization. PET/CT shows relapse in 14 pts. PET/CT > CT for detection of intrahepatic recurrence
Higashi et al,[109] 2010	R	67	6 RFA	Primary CHC	—	1 mo	16 false negative/67 local therapies
Kim et al,[51] 2012	R	31/45	2 RFA, 40 TACE	Primary CHC	—	—	Visual analysis > SUVmax/SUV normal liver
Sahin et al,[110] 2012	R	—	Laparoscopic RFA	M + CLM	—	104 PET/CT during follow-up	PET/CT > CECT Additional information in 25% cases
Chen et al,[111] 2013	R	28/33	RFA	Primary, M+	17/33 residual or recurrent tumor	—	—
Nielsen et al,[82,112] 2013	R	79/179	RFA	—	30 relapses at 1 y	57 PET at 6 mo	—

(continued on next page)

Table 2
(continued)

Author (Ref), Year	R/P/M	No. of Pts./Lesions	Technique	Cancer Type	Local Control	Timing of PET/CT	Remarks
Wang et al,[113] 2013	—	—	16 RFA± hepatectomy	Primary	—	—	PET/CT > CEUS
Kornberg et al,[114] 2013	R	—	63 TACE 8 RFA	—	50% necrosis at explant pathology	Workup After local treatment before liver transplantation	If PET + before transplant, worse prognosis
Nielsen et al,[49] 2014	P	20	RFA, MW	M+	—	Every 3 mo	PET and MRI compared with PET/CT
Vandenbroucke et al,[115] 2014	R	20/45	RFA	M+	—	—	Pattern I: no FDG uptake Pattern II: rimlike pattern Pattern III: peripheral nodule. If > 1 cm VPP = 100%
Zheng et al,[116] 2014	M	155	RFA	—	—	—	7 studies

Abbreviations: AFP, α-fetoprotein level; CRY, cryotherapy; M, meta-analysis; M+, metastases; MWA, microwaves; NA, not available; NPV, negative predictive value; P, prospective; R, retrospective; TACE, transarterial chemoembolization.

for PET/CT timing, but very early PET/CT at 24 hours or 1 week is not very useful and 3 to 6 months for first postablation PET/CT evaluation is a good compromise. It is repeated every 3 months the first year because local progression is more frequent the first year after thermal ablation and then every 6 months.

Because the sensitivity of MRI as a detection method for small intrahepatic lesions is high and FDG-PET is able to visualize enhanced metabolism at the ablation site, FDG-PET-MRI could potentially improve the accuracy of detection of progressive disease and thus allow an early re-treatment relapse after thermal ablation.[49]

Liver Primary Cancer

Primary liver carcinoma, hepatocellular carcinoma (HCC), is fifth in cancer incidence in the world and the third leading cause of cancer-related death. Hepatic resection and transplantation are the optimal treatments; however, less than 20% are surgical candidates, and thermal ablation is used more often. Radiofrequency is the most frequent thermal ablation option chosen.

PET/CT is sensitive in detecting residual or relapse malignancy after thermal ablation in scarred liver disease but its limit is relatively low in sensibility attributable to the degree of glucose-6-phosphatase in HCC. If PET/CT is used for response evaluation, a pretreatment PET/CT should be performed to check if the lesions are FDG-avid. If they are not, a negative posttreatment PET/CT could result in a false negative result.

Hapatocellular carcinoma has variable 18F-FDG uptake and in the Paudyal[50] study, the pre-RFA standard uptake value (SUV) was higher in poorly or moderately differentiated HCC than in well-differentiated cases.

Only 4 studies are dedicated to PET/CT in primary liver cancer treated by thermal ablation. In one study, 2 RFA-treated HCCs show a rim-shaped FDG uptake on the PET/CT performed 1 day after RFA.[51]

Kidney Malignancies

RFA and cryotherapy are being increasingly used for the treatment of primary or secondary renal carcinoma. In a systematic review, Katsanos and colleagues[52] have shown that thermal ablation of small renal masses produces oncologic outcomes similar to surgical nephrectomy and is associated with significantly lower overall complication rates and a significantly smaller decline in renal function. Because of the low Glut-1 expression in primary renal cancer, PET/CT is rarely used for workup or response evaluation, and there are no articles describing use of PET/CT for thermal ablation evaluation.

Skeletal and Soft Tissue Diseases

There are very few studies describing thermal ablation in primary bone tumors because they are very aggressive tumors and thermal ablation is rarely used for primary bone tumors. However, thermal ablation can be useful to treat metastases, mainly lung metastases from soft tissue and bone tumors.[29] In contrast, thermal ablation is used more often for treating osteolytic bone metastases.

Bone Metastases

Bone metastases are common in many advanced cancer types and are a frequent source of clinical morbidity. About 30% of all malignant tumors induce bone metastases, particularly breast, lung, prostate, and kidney cancers, but also anaplastic, poorly differentiated, follicular or onco-cytic thyroid carcinomas. Treatment of bone metastases has 3 goals: pain relief, maintaining mobility, and improving quality of life and survival. Until recently, the treatment options were surgery,[53] radiation therapy, and systemic therapy, but more thermal ablation with or without cementoplasty is used because of the low morbidity, efficacy to these goals, repeatability, and short hospitalization.[54] For small tumors (less than 3 cm), radiofrequency[55] can be used, but for larger tumors, cryotherapy is a good choice, even though it is an expensive technique, because an interventional radiologist can place several parallel needles and treat very large metastases while preserving the adjacent structure given the visibility of the ice-ball (**Fig. 3**) on the CT.[56–59] Treatment response is very challenging in bone lesions because RECIST criteria are often not applicable and PET/CT can be used for planning when a retreatment is warranted and if the bone metastases are FDG-avid. **Fig. 3** is an example of PET/CT follow-up after cryotherapy.

Benign Bone Tumors

Thermal ablation is used more often for the treatment of osteoid osteoma,[60] which requires ablation of the nidus, for osteoblastoma, or for aneurysmal cysts.[61] Laser may be used for osteoid osteomas with success in 97% of cases.[62] Cryotherapy can be useful for treating large, benign, painful tumors, and PET/CT is useful for response evaluation if the lesions are FDG-avid as in 3 case reports of osteoblastoma or osteoid osteomas.[63]

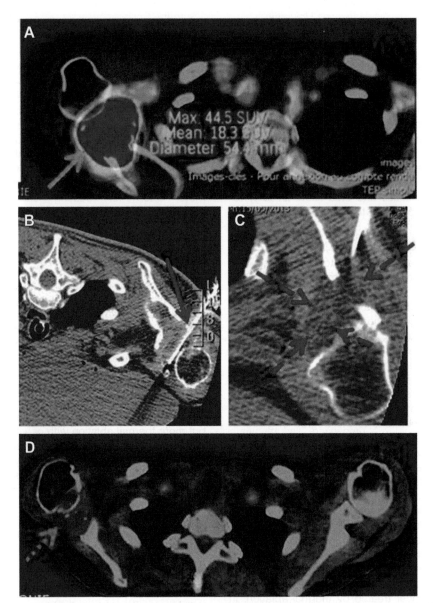

Fig. 3. True-negative PET/CT after cryotherapy for bone metastasis. A 48-year-old woman with very painful large unique bone scapula metastasis from iodine refractory oncocytic thyroid carcinoma. The patient refused extensive surgery. Radiotherapy + 2 cryotherapies + cementoplasty were performed. Probe is percutaneously introduced into the osteolytic lesion (*B, red arrow*). The iceball is monitored by CT scan (*C, red dashed arrows*). PET/CT before cryotherapy (*A, blue arrow*) shows very intense FDG uptake (SUVmax = 44.5). After 3 months, there is no more FDG uptake (*D, blue dashed arrow*). The thyroglobulin biomarker for differentiated thyroid carcinoma has decreased from 17,450 to 1.7 ng/mL, which is in favor of a good response; no local progression 4 years later.

Complications of Thermal Ablation in Soft Tissue or Bone Lesions

Muscular injury around the cryoablation is commonly observed but rarely symptomatic and can be treated by anti-inflammatory drugs.[64] This inflammation may be a cause of false positive PET/CT.

Thyroid Cancer

Differentiated thyroid cancer is a slowly evolving disease with potential patients' long life expectancy.[65,66] They are treated by surgery and radioiodine if there is a high relapse risk, but distant metastases occur in 10% to 15% of the patients,[67] with lung and bone being the most affected organs. Lung metastases are usually asymptomatic, thus being discovered incidentally during routine radiological follow-up. If they are responding to radioiodine, the survival matches survival for nonmetastatic patients.[68] In contrast, bone metastases are often symptomatic and thus frequently cause pain, swelling, fractures, neural compression, and functional deficits.[69] Farooki and colleagues[70] have shown that when a first bone metastasis occurs, skeletal-related events are more likely to occur. Therefore, symptoms from bone metastases may severely alter patients' quality of life. According to the American Thyroid Association Guidelines on Thyroid Nodules and Differentiated Thyroid Cancer, metastatic bone disease is treated with Iodine-131 therapy, external beam radiation, and surgery.[71] When lung or bone metastases are iodine refractory,[72] chemotherapy is ineffective, and local thermal ablation may be considered when they are slowly growing (RECIST progression >1 year) even if there is no strong evidence for that.[73] PET/CT is rarely positive in differentiated carcinoma, but when it is, there is a poor prognostic factor. In these cases, PET/CT can be useful for follow-up after local treatments. **Fig. 4**

is an example of a good result of liver and lung thermal ablation in an iodine refractory oncocytic carcinoma. **Fig. 3** shows a very favorable result after cryotherapy for large unique scapular bone metastases from thyroid oncocytic carcinoma.

Breast Cancer

Thermal ablation techniques, such as RFA or stereotactic interstitial laser therapy,[73] are under investigation, especially in older women,[74] but usefulness of PET/CT is not demonstrated in small lesions. Nair and colleagues[73] have shown in 4 patients that PET/CT results and histology were both in favor of necrosis. Noguchi and colleagues[75] used thermal ablation combined with sentinel node ablation in T1N0M0 tumors. They used PET/CT for the follow-up at 6 months and every year afterward, but they do not describe in how many people PET/CT was performed and what were the results.

REAL-TIME GUIDING THERMAL ABLATION

Real-time guiding thermal ablation is under investigation.[76–78] However, there is an advantage to

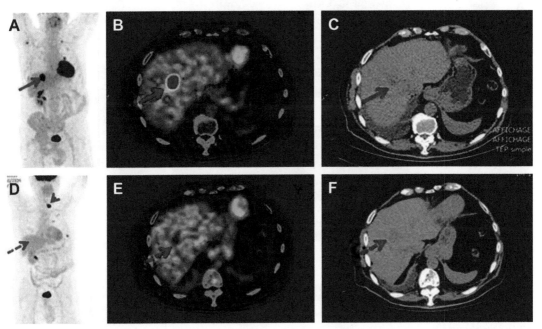

Fig. 4. True-negative PET/CT after RFA for a thyroid liver metastasis. A 68-year-old man with pT3N0M0 oncocytic thyroid carcinoma; 3.5 y after initial diagnosis, he developed many lung metastases, which were treated by RFA, and one unique liver metastasis treated by RFA 7 years after initial diagnosis. (*A–C*) PET/CT performed before RFA shows the liver metastasis (*red arrows*). It is more easily visualized on PET image (*B*) because of the intense FDG uptake than on the CT image (*C*). (*D–F*) PET/CT performed 6 months after liver RFA shows complete remission of the liver metastasis (*red dashed arrow*), but an appearance of a new neck relapse (*red arrowhead*), which was treated by surgery. He also had other lung RFA and is now 81 years old in complete clinical and biological remission (thyroglobulin is 0.4 ng/mL) with very good quality of life.

target the more aggressive lesion, but because of radioprotection problems, there is not yet a standard.

LIMITS OF 18F-FLUORODEOXYGLUCOSE PET/COMPUTED TOMOGRAPHY

18F-FDG PET/CT visualizes increased glucose metabolism, which is common in cancer cells, but in some cases, they are not 18F-FDG-avid. If a lesion treated by thermal ablation is not 18F-FDG-avid, PET/CT cannot be used for post-treatment evaluation. This can be observed for some slowly metastases cancers: mucinous colonic cancer and some metastases from differentiated or medullary thyroid carcinoma. In some cases, medullary thyroid carcinoma or neuroendocrine metastases, and other radionuclides,

like I124[79] or fluorodopa[80] or 11C-5-tryptophan,[81] can be used but are not always used in a routine context.

False Negative Follow-Up Results

If a preablation PET/CT has shown the FDG-avidity of the lesion, there are very few false negative results for lung metastases.[40] For primary lung cancer or primary or secondary liver cancers, it can persist as some residual cells at the periphery of ablated zone are not visible on the early PET/CT, which may recur later.

The resolution of FDG-PET/CT is approximately 7 mm, and a very small relapse developed from some residual viable cells after thermal ablation may be not visualized on PET/CT (**Fig. 5**). As mentioned by Nielsen and colleagues,[82] if there

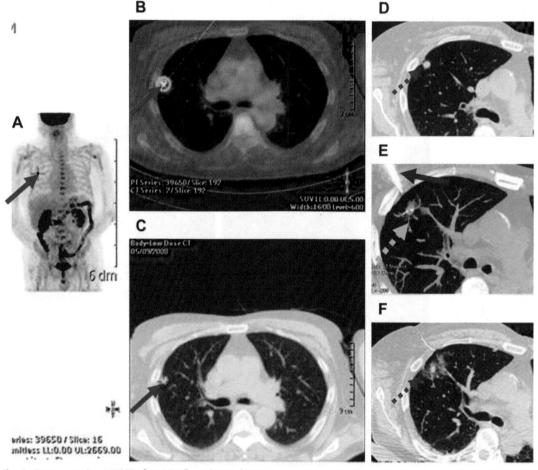

Fig. 5. True-negative PET/CT after RFA for primary lung cancer. A 75-year-old man with inoperable T1aN0M0 primary lung cancer. (*A, red arrow*) Maximum intensity projection (MIP). (*B, red arrow*) PET shows high uptake in the nodule. (*C, red arrow*) CT of the PET/CT. (*D, dashed red arrow*) Nodule just before RFA; the patient is positioned for good access to the lesion. (*E*) Needle is percutaneously introduced (*dotted blue arrow*) into the center of the nodule and the prongs are deployed (*dashed blue arrow*). (*F*) On the post-RFA CT, there is a large ground-glass opacity around the dense lesion (*dotted red arrow*).

is a new small, hypodense lesion on contrast-enhanced CT, even if there is no FDG uptake on PET/CT, it should be considered suspicious of local relapse.

False Positive Results

Specificity is low because of inflammatory changes after thermal ablation. For example, in a large prospective study dedicated to lung metastases treated by RFA, the specificity is only 66.3%, but the predictive positive value is different according the image pattern.[40] Three types of images were associated with local recurrence: moderate or high uptake far from the pleura, rim plus nodular uptake in or beside the rim, and cavitation.[40] Before re-treating a lesion with FDG uptake, it is recommended to look at the CT images if there is an increase in the size of the lesion compared with the postablation CT; if it is doubtful, close follow-up or biopsy should be performed (**Fig. 6**).

True Positive Results

PET/CT true positive results are often earlier than positive CT (**Fig. 7**).

True Negative Results

PET/CT true negative results are very frequent and useful (**Figs. 4** and **8**). In the authors' prospective study about radiofrequency for lung metastases, the negative predictive value of PET/CT was as high as 98.3%.[40]

SUMMARY

Thermal ablation is used more often in oncology for primary and secondary cancer, but also to destroy benign tumors. PET/CT plays an important role in the follow-up to detect residual viable tissue and then to detect early a relapse that can be re-treated by thermal ablation or other means. Postablation aspects must be well known by the specialist in charge of image interpretation. He has to know not only the metabolic aspect but also the CT aspects, which are very different from the usual aspects seen after other treatments, like chemotherapy.[83]

All studies are concordant to conclude that PET/CT is a useful tool for early recognition of incomplete tumor destruction after thermal ablation

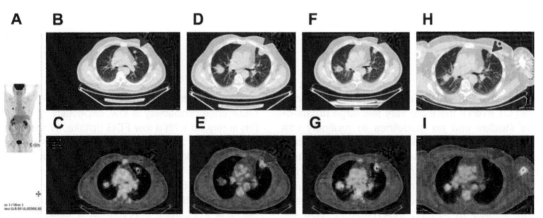

Fig. 6. False-positive PET/CT after RFA for colorectal lung metastasis. (*A*) PET/CT before RFA and MIP before RFA. (*B*, *C*) Transaxial images of PET/CT before RFA (*red arrow*). Two nodules were treated by RFA. (*D*, *E*) PET/CT done 1 month after RFA images shows on the CT (*D*) that the left nodule is larger than before RFA and on the PET an incomplete rimlike image with faint FDG uptake (SUVmax 2.6; it was 10.3 before RFA) near the pleura interpreted as normal postablation aspect (*red dashed arrow*). (*F*, *G*) PET/CT 3 months after RFA (*red dotted arrow*). On the CT, the nodule size has decreased, but on the PET there is again an intense FDG uptake (SUVmax = 6.6) in the left lesion; this was suspicious of a local relapse. Biopsy was performed, but no malignant cells were found; only inflammatory cells were observed. (*H*, *I*) PET/CT 1 year after RFA (*red arrowhead*). On the CT, it persists as a scar, but on the PET image, there was no FDG uptake in the left nodule (SUVmax = 0.9).

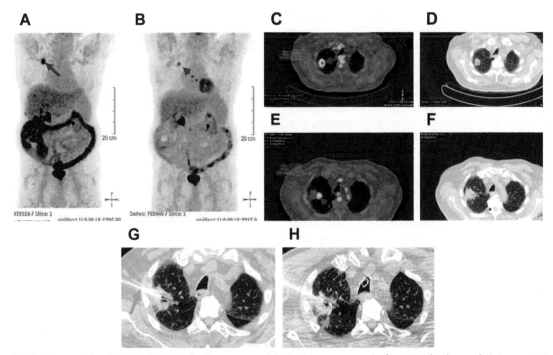

Fig. 7. True-positive PET/CT after RFA for lung cancer. (*A, C, D*) Lung cancer before RFA (*red arrow*): intense FDG uptake in the right lung nodule. (*A*) Maximum intensity projection (MIP); (*C, D*) PET/CT images. (*G*) RFA procedure; needle (*green arrow*) is percutaneously introduced into the tumor; then prongs are deployed (*H, green arrow*). (*B, E, F*) Lung cancer 3 months after RFA: PET/CT at 3 months shows a local relapse 6 months after lung RFA (*red dotted arrow*); at the periphery of a dense irregular nodule, there is a small spot of intense FDG uptake. (*B*) MIP; (*E, F*) PET/CT images.

whatever the site. It also detects recurrence earlier than CT even if there are very few large prospective studies and no guidelines to routinely use PET/CT. Despite these limits, it could be a good adjunct to other imaging modalities to detect recurrence early and re-treat them by another thermal ablation or by other means (SBRT or surgery). No standardized regimen or diagnostic criteria with respect to PET/CT interpretation have yet been proposed in the literature. However, in this literature review, some consensus points must be underlined. It seems good timing to perform follow-up by PET/CT at 3–9 months and then every 6 months because recurrences are generally observed during the first year after thermal ablation. The image interpretation is easy when there is a total photopenia. When there is a rim-shaped

uptake, due to inflammation or hyperemia, the recurrence probability is low, especially when the rim is regular with a low FDG uptake. When there is an irregular zone at the periphery of the ablated zone with a high FDG uptake, the predictive value of recurrence is very high and close follow-up or biopsy must be done to confirm the recurrence and re-treat the lesion. When the ablated zone become FDG-avid, it could be a false positive case linked to delayed inflammation, and the lesion size on the CT or the enhancement on a CECT must be checked.

Prospective studies are needed to demonstrate that use of PET/CT follow-up for early detection of relapses, which permits early re-treatment, may improve overall survival in different types of primary or secondary cancer.

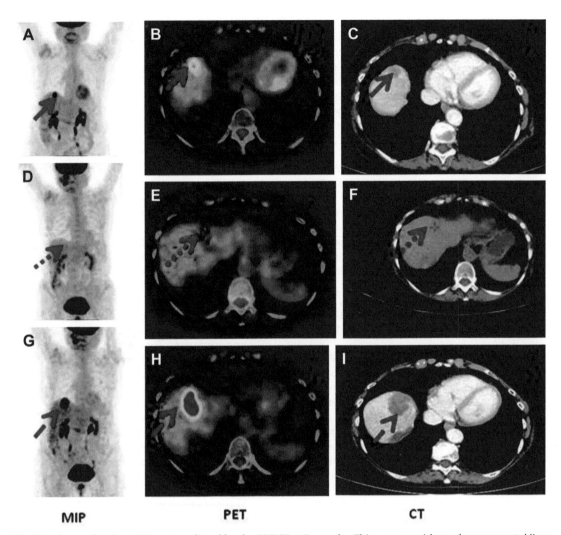

MIP   PET   CT

Fig. 8. Relapse after liver RFA not predicted by the PET/CT at 5 months. This woman with synchronous rectal liver metastases was treated by primary chemotherapy; because of persistent liver metastasis 1.5 months later, RFA was performed. (*A–C*) Liver nodule before RFA (*red arrow*). The PET/CT performed before RFA shows an intense FDG uptake on the MIP (*A*) and the PET (*B*). On the contrast-enhanced CT, the nodule is hypodense (*C*). The follow-up PET/CT 5 months after RFA was normal (*D–F*) with a total photopenic area on the PET (*D, E, red dotted arrows*) and a hypodense aspect on the CT (*F, red dotted arrows*), but on the PET/CT done 3 months later, there is a relapse with intense FDG uptake (*G, H, red dashed arrows*) and increased size of the hypodense lesion on the CT (*I, red dashed arrow*).

REFERENCES

1. Mijnhout GS, Hooft L, van Tulder MW, et al. How to perform a comprehensive search for FDG-PET literature. Eur J Nucl Med 2000;27(1):91–7.
2. Mijnhout GS, Riphagen II, Hoekstra OS. Update of the FDG PET search strategy. Nucl Med Commun 2004;25(12):1187–9.
3. Dupuy DE. Image-guided thermal ablation of lung malignancies. Radiology 2011;260(3):633–55.
4. Palussiere J, Pellerin-Guignard A, Descat E, et al. Radiofrequency ablation of bone tumours. Diagn Interv Imaging 2012;93(9):660–4.
5. Haissaguerre M, Saoudi N. Role of catheter ablation for supraventricular tachyarrhythmias, with emphasis on atrial flutter and atrial tachycardia. Curr Opin Cardiol 1994;9(1):40–52.
6. Dickfeld T, Lei P, Dilsizian V, et al. Integration of three-dimensional scar maps for ventricular tachycardia ablation with positron emission tomography-computed tomography. JACC Cardiovasc Imaging 2008;1(1):73–82.
7. Dickfeld T, Kocher C. The role of integrated PET-CT scar maps for guiding ventricular tachycardia ablations. Curr Cardiol Rep 2008;10(2):149–57.

8. Fahmy TS, Wazni OM, Jaber WA, et al. Integration of positron emission tomography/computed tomography with electroanatomical mapping: a novel approach for ablation of scar-related ventricular tachycardia. Heart Rhythm 2008;5(11):1538–45.

9. Thachil A, Christopher J, Sastry BK, et al. Monomorphic ventricular tachycardia and mediastinal adenopathy due to granulomatous infiltration in patients with preserved ventricular function. J Am Coll Cardiol 2011;58(1):48–55.

10. Simon CJ, Dupuy DE, Mayo-Smith WW. Microwave ablation: principles and applications. Radiographics 2005;25(Suppl 1):S69–83.

11. Gangi A. Interventional musculoskeletal radiology. Eur Radiol 2002;12(6):1235–6.

12. Buy X, Basile A, Bierry G, et al. Saline-infused bipolar radiofrequency ablation of high-risk spinal and paraspinal neoplasms. AJR Am J Roentgenol 2006;186(5 Suppl):S322–6.

13. Goldberg SN, Gazelle GS, Compton CC, et al. Radiofrequency tissue ablation in the rabbit lung: efficacy and complications. Acad Radiol 1995;2(9):776–84.

14. Ohira T, Okuma T, Matsuoka T, et al. FDG-MicroPET and diffusion-weighted MR image evaluation of early changes after radiofrequency ablation in implanted VX2 tumors in rabbits. Cardiovasc Intervent Radiol 2009;32(1):114–20.

15. Okuma T, Matsuoka T, Okamura T, et al. 18F-FDG small-animal PET for monitoring the therapeutic effect of CT-guided radiofrequency ablation on implanted VX2 lung tumors in rabbits. J Nucl Med 2006;47(8):1351–8.

16. Tominaga J, Miyachi H, Takase K, et al. Time-related changes in computed tomographic appearance and pathologic findings after radiofrequency ablation of the rabbit lung: preliminary experimental study. J Vasc Interv Radiol 2005;16(12):1719–26.

17. Vogt FM, Antoch G, Veit P, et al. Morphologic and functional changes in nontumorous liver tissue after radiofrequency ablation in an in vivo model: comparison of 18F-FDG PET/CT, MRI, ultrasound, and CT. J Nucl Med 2007;48(11):1836–44.

18. Yamamoto A, Nakamura K, Matsuoka T, et al. Radiofrequency ablation in a porcine lung model: correlation between CT and histopathologic findings. AJR Am J Roentgenol 2005;185(5):1299–306.

19. Kashima M, Yamakado K, Takaki H, et al. Complications after 1000 lung radiofrequency ablation sessions in 420 patients: a single center's experiences. AJR Am J Roentgenol 2011;197(4):W576–80.

20. Alberti N, Frulio N, Trillaud H, et al. Pulmonary aspergilloma in a cavity formed after percutaneous radiofrequency ablation. Cardiovasc Intervent Radiol 2014;37(2):537–40.

21. Hiraki T, Gobara H, Fujiwara H, et al. Lung cancer ablation: complications. Semin Intervent Radiol 2013;30(2):169–75.

22. Palussiere J, Marcet B, Descat E, et al. Lung tumors treated with percutaneous radiofrequency ablation: computed tomography imaging follow-up. Cardiovasc Intervent Radiol 2010;34(5):989–97.

23. Eisenhauer EA, Therasse P, Bogaerts J, et al. New response evaluation criteria in solid tumours: revised RECIST guideline (version 1.1). Eur J Cancer 2009;45(2):228–47.

24. Goto T, Izumi Y, Nakatsuka S, et al. Percutaneous cryoablation as a salvage therapy for local recurrence of lung cancer. Ann Thorac Surg 2012;94(2):e31–3.

25. Chua TC, Sarkar A, Saxena A, et al. Long-term outcome of image-guided percutaneous radiofrequency ablation of lung metastases: an open-labeled prospective trial of 148 patients. Ann Oncol 2010;21(10):2017–22.

26. de Baere T, Auperin A, Deschamps F, et al. Radiofrequency ablation is a valid treatment option for lung metastases: Experience in 566 patients with 1037 metastases. Ann Oncol 2015;26(5):987–91.

27. Gillams AR, Lees WR. Five-year survival following radiofrequency ablation of small, solitary, hepatic colorectal metastases. J Vasc Interv Radiol 2008;19(5):712–7.

28. Koelblinger C, Strauss S, Gillams A. Outcome after radiofrequency ablation of sarcoma lung metastases. Cardiovasc Intervent Radiol 2014;37(1):147–53.

29. Palussiere J, Italiano A, Descat E, et al. Sarcoma lung metastases treated with percutaneous radiofrequency ablation: results from 29 patients. Ann Surg Oncol 2011;18(13):3771–7.

30. Hiraki T, Gobara H, Iishi T, et al. Percutaneous radiofrequency ablation for clinical stage I non-small cell lung cancer: results in 20 nonsurgical candidates. J Thorac Cardiovasc Surg 2007;134(5):1306–12.

31. Lanuti M, Sharma A, Digumarthy SR, et al. Radiofrequency ablation for treatment of medically inoperable stage I non-small cell lung cancer. J Thorac Cardiovasc Surg 2009;137(1):160–6.

32. Pennathur A, Luketich JD, Abbas G, et al. Radiofrequency ablation for the treatment of stage I non-small cell lung cancer in high-risk patients. J Thorac Cardiovasc Surg 2007;134(4):857–64.

33. Simon CJ, Dupuy DE, DiPetrillo TA, et al. Pulmonary radiofrequency ablation: long-term safety and efficacy in 153 patients. Radiology 2007;243(1):268–75.

34. Crabtree T, Puri V, Timmerman R, et al. Treatment of stage I lung cancer in high-risk and inoperable patients: comparison of prospective clinical trials using stereotactic body radiotherapy (RTOG 0236),

sublobar resection (ACOSOG Z4032), and radio-frequency ablation (ACOSOG Z4033). J Thorac Cardiovasc Surg 2013;145(3):692–9.

35. Lanuti M, Sharma A, Willers H, et al. Radiofrequency ablation for stage I non-small cell lung cancer: management of locoregional recurrence. Ann Thorac Surg 2012;93(3):921–7.

36. Acksteiner C, Steinke K. Percutaneous microwave ablation for early-stage non-small cell lung cancer (NSCLC) in the elderly: a promising outlook. J Med Imaging Radiat Oncol 2015;59(1):82–90.

37. Giraud P, Antoine M, Larrouy A, et al. Evaluation of microscopic tumor extension in non-small-cell lung cancer for three-dimensional conformal radiotherapy planning. Int J Radiat Oncol Biol Phys 2000;48(4):1015–24.

38. Beland MD, Wasser EJ, Mayo-Smith WW, et al. Primary non-small cell lung cancer: review of frequency, location, and time of recurrence after radiofrequency ablation. Radiology 2010;254(1):301–7.

39. Abtin FG, Eradat J, Gutierrez AJ, et al. Radiofrequency ablation of lung tumors: imaging features of the postablation zone. Radiographics 2012; 32(4):947–69.

40. Bonichon F, Palussiere J, Godbert Y, et al. Diagnostic accuracy of F-FDG PET/CT for assessing response to radiofrequency ablation treatment in lung metastases: a multicentre prospective study. Eur J Nucl Med Mol Imaging 2013;40:1817–27.

41. Deandreis D, Leboulleux S, Dromain C, et al. Role of FDG PET/CT and chest CT in the follow-up of lung lesions treated with radiofrequency ablation. Radiology 2011;258(1):270–6.

42. Purandare NC, Rangarajan V, Shah SA, et al. Therapeutic response to radiofrequency ablation of neoplastic lesions: FDG PET/CT findings. Radiographics 2011;31(1):201–13.

43. Singnurkar A, Solomon SB, Gonen M, et al. 18F-FDG PET/CT for the prediction and detection of local recurrence after radiofrequency ablation of malignant lung lesions. J Nucl Med 2010;51(12): 1833–40.

44. Bala MM, Riemsma RP, Wolff R, et al. Cryotherapy for liver metastases. Cochrane Database Syst Rev 2013;(6):CD009058.

45. Bala MM, Riemsma RP, Wolff R, et al. Microwave coagulation for liver metastases. Cochrane Database Syst Rev 2013;(10):CD010163.

46. Wong SL, Mangu PB, Choti MA, et al. American Society of Clinical Oncology 2009 clinical evidence review on radiofrequency ablation of hepatic metastases from colorectal cancer. J Clin Oncol 2010;28(3):493–508.

47. Oshowo A, Gillams A, Harrison E, et al. Comparison of resection and radiofrequency ablation for treatment of solitary colorectal liver metastases. Br J Surg 2003;90(10):1240–3.

48. Berber E, Pelley R, Siperstein AE. Predictors of survival after radiofrequency thermal ablation of colorectal cancer metastases to the liver: a prospective study. J Clin Oncol 2005;23(7):1358–64.

49. Nielsen K, Scheffer HJ, Pieters IC, et al. The use of PET-MRI in the follow-up after radiofrequency- and microwave ablation of colorectal liver metastases. BMC Med Imaging 2014;14(1):27.

50. Paudyal B, Oriuchi N, Paudyal P, et al. Early diagnosis of recurrent hepatocellular carcinoma with 18F-FDG PET after radiofrequency ablation therapy. Oncol Rep 2007;18(6):1469–73.

51. Kim SH, Won KS, Choi BW, et al. Usefulness of F-18 FDG PET/CT in the evaluation of early treatment response after interventional therapy for hepatocellular carcinoma. Nucl Med Mol Imaging 2012; 46(2):102–10.

52. Katsanos K, Mailli L, Krokidis M, et al. Systematic review and meta-analysis of thermal ablation versus surgical nephrectomy for small renal tumours. Cardiovasc Intervent Radiol 2014;37(2):427–37.

53. Agarwal MG, Nayak P. Management of skeletal metastases: an orthopaedic surgeon's guide. Indian J Orthop 2015;49(1):83–100.

54. Sabharwal T, Katsanos K, Buy X, et al. Image-guided ablation therapy of bone tumors. Semin Ultrasound CT MR 2009;30(2):78–90.

55. Dupuy DE, Liu D, Hartfeil D, et al. Percutaneous radiofrequency ablation of painful osseous metastases: a multicenter American College of Radiology Imaging Network trial. Cancer 2010;116(4): 989–97.

56. Callstrom MR, Kurup AN. Percutaneous ablation for bone and soft tissue metastases–why cryoablation? Skeletal Radiol 2009;38(9):835–9.

57. Callstrom MR, Charboneau JW. Image-guided palliation of painful metastases using percutaneous ablation. Tech Vasc Interv Radiol 2007; 10(2):120–31.

58. Callstrom MR, Atwell TD, Charboneau JW, et al. Painful metastases involving bone: percutaneous image-guided cryoablation–prospective trial interim analysis. Radiology 2006;241(2):572–80.

59. Callstrom MR, Charboneau JW, Goetz MP, et al. Image-guided ablation of painful metastatic bone tumors: a new and effective approach to a difficult problem. Skeletal Radiol 2006;35(1):1–15.

60. Moser T, Giacomelli MC, Clavert JM, et al. Image-guided laser ablation of osteoid osteoma in pediatric patients. J Pediatr Orthop 2008;28(2):265–70.

61. Tsoumakidou G, Too CW, Garnon J, et al. Treatment of a spinal aneurysmal bone cyst using combined image-guided cryoablation and cementoplasty. Skeletal Radiol 2015;44(2):285–9.

62. Gangi A, Alizadeh H, Wong L, et al. Osteoid osteoma: percutaneous laser ablation and follow-up in 114 patients. Radiology 2007;242(1):293–301.

63. Imperiale A, Moser T, Ben-Sellem D, et al. Osteo-blastoma and osteoid osteoma: morphofunctional characterization by MRI and dynamic F-18 FDG PET/CT before and after radiofrequency ablation. Clin Nucl Med 2009;34(3):184–8.

64. Bing F, Garnon J, Tsoumakidou G, et al. Imaging-guided percutaneous cryotherapy of bone and soft-tissue tumors: what is the impact on the muscles around the ablation site? AJR Am J Roentgenol 2014;202(6):1361–5.

65. Schlumberger MJ. Papillary and follicular thyroid carcinoma. N Engl J Med 1998;338(5):297–306.

66. Sherman SI. Thyroid carcinoma. Lancet 2003; 361(9356):501–11.

67. Muresan MM, Olivier P, Leclere J, et al. Bone metastases from differentiated thyroid carcinoma. Endocr Relat Cancer 2008;15(1):37–49.

68. Durante C, Haddy N, Baudin E, et al. Long-term outcome of 444 patients with distant metastases from papillary and follicular thyroid carcinoma: benefits and limits of radioiodine therapy. J Clin Endocrinol Metab 2006;91(8):2892–9.

69. Schlumberger M, Challeton C, de Vathaire F, et al. Radioactive iodine treatment and external radiotherapy for lung and bone metastases from thyroid carcinoma. J Nucl Med 1996;37(4): 598–605.

70. Farooki A, Leung V, Tala H, et al. Skeletal-related events due to bone metastases from differentiated thyroid cancer. J Clin Endocrinol Metab 2012;97(7): 2433–9.

71. Cooper DS, Doherty GM, Haugen BR, et al. Revised American Thyroid Association management guidelines for patients with thyroid nodules and differentiated thyroid cancer. Thyroid 2009; 19(11):1167–214.

72. Schlumberger M, Brose M, Elisei R, et al. Definition and management of radioactive iodine-refractory differentiated thyroid cancer. Lancet Diabetes Endocrinol 2014;2(5):356–8.

73. Nair N, Ali A, Dowlatshahi K, et al. Positron emission tomography with fluorine-18 fluorodeoxyglucose to evaluate response of early breast carcinoma treated with stereotaxic interstitial laser therapy. Clin Nucl Med 2000;25(7):505–7.

74. Palussiere J, Henriques C, Mauriac L, et al. Radiofrequency ablation as a substitute for surgery in elderly patients with nonresected breast cancer: pilot study with long-term outcomes. Radiology 2012;264(2):597–605.

75. Noguchi M, Motoyoshi A, Earashi M, et al. Long-term outcome of breast cancer patients treated with radiofrequency ablation. Eur J Surg Oncol 2012;38(11):1036–42.

76. Schoellnast H, Larson SM, Nehmeh SA, et al. Radiofrequency ablation of non-small-cell carcinoma of the lung under real-time FDG PET CT guidance. Cardiovasc Intervent Radiol 2010;34(Suppl 2): S182–5.

77. Krucker J, Xu S, Venkatesan A, et al. Clinical utility of real-time fusion guidance for biopsy and ablation. J Vasc Interv Radiol 2011;22(4):515–24.

78. Venkatesan AM, Kadoury S, Abi-Jaoudeh N, et al. Real-time FDG PET guidance during biopsies and radiofrequency ablation using multimodality fusion with electromagnetic navigation. Radiology 2011; 260(3):848–56.

79. Freudenberg LS, Antoch G, Jentzen W, et al. Value of (124)I-PET/CT in staging of patients with differentiated thyroid cancer. Eur Radiol 2004;14(11): 2092–8.

80. Treglia G, Stefanelli A, Castaldi P, et al. A standardized dual-phase 18F-DOPA PET/CT protocol in the detection of medullary thyroid cancer. Nucl Med Commun 2013;34(2):185–6.

81. Norlen O, Nilsson A, Krause J, et al. 11C-5-hydroxytryptophan positron emission tomography after radiofrequency ablation of neuroendocrine tumor liver metastases. Nucl Med Biol 2012; 39(6):883–90.

82. Nielsen K, van Tilborg AA, Scheffer HJ, et al. PET-CT after radiofrequency ablation of colorectal liver metastases: suggestions for timing and image interpretation. Eur J Radiol 2013; 82(12):2169–75.

83. Basu S, Kumar R, Ranade R. Assessment of treatment response using PET. PET Clin 2015; 10(1):9–26.

84. Kang S, Luo R, Liao W, et al. Single group study to evaluate the feasibility and complications of radiofrequency ablation and usefulness of post treatment position emission tomography in lung tumours. World J Surg Oncol 2004;2(1):30.

85. Hataji O, Yamakado K, Nakatsuka A, et al. Radiological and pathological correlation of lung malignant tumors treated with percutaneous radiofrequency ablation. Intern Med 2005;44(8): 865–9.

86. Okuma T, Okamura T, Matsuoka T, et al. Fluorine-18-fluorodeoxyglucose positron emission tomography for assessment of patients with unresectable recurrent or metastatic lung cancers after CT-guided radiofrequency ablation: preliminary results. Ann Nucl Med 2006;20(2):115–21.

87. Higaki F, Okumura Y, Sato S, et al. Preliminary retrospective investigation of FDG-PET/CT timing in follow-up of ablated lung tumor. Ann Nucl Med 2008;22(3):157–63.

88. Harada S, Sato S, Suzuki E, et al. The usefulness of pre-radiofrequency ablation SUVmax in 18F-FDG PET/CT to predict the risk of a local recurrence of malignant lung tumors after lung radiofrequency ablation. Acta Med Okayama 2011; 65(6):395–402.

89. Yoo DC, Dupuy DE, Hillman SL, et al. Radiofrequency ablation of medically inoperable stage IA non-small cell lung cancer: are early posttreatment PET findings predictive of treatment outcome? AJR Am J Roentgenol 2011;197(2):334–40.

90. Schoellnast H, Deodhar A, Hsu M, et al. Recurrent non-small cell lung cancer: evaluation of CT-guided radiofrequency ablation as salvage therapy. Acta Radiol 2012;53(8):893–9.

91. Alafate A, Shinya T, Okumura Y, et al. The maximum standardized uptake value is more reliable than size measurement in early follow-up to evaluate potential pulmonary malignancies following radiofrequency ablation. Acta Med Okayama 2013;67(2):105–12.

92. Gadaleta CD, Solbiati L, Mattioli V, et al. Unresectable lung malignancy: combination therapy with segmental pulmonary arterial chemoembolization with drug-eluting microspheres and radiofrequency ablation in 17 patients. Radiology 2013;267(2):627–37.

93. Kodama H, Yamakado K, Takaki H, et al. Impact of 18F-FDG-PET/CT on treatment strategy in colorectal cancer lung metastasis before lung radiofrequency ablation. Nucl Med Commun 2013;34(7): 689–93.

94. Sharma A, Lanuti M, He W, et al. Increase in fluorodeoxyglucose positron emission tomography activity following complete radiofrequency ablation of lung tumors. J Comput Assist Tomogr 2013;37(1):9–14.

95. Higuchi M, Honjo H, Shigihara T, et al. A phase II study of radiofrequency ablation therapy for thoracic malignancies with evaluation by FDG-PET. J Cancer Res Clin Oncol 2014;140(11):1957–63.

96. Langenhoff BS, Oyen WJ, Jager GJ, et al. Efficacy of fluorine-18-deoxyglucose positron emission tomography in detecting tumor recurrence after local ablative therapy for liver metastases: a prospective study. J Clin Oncol 2002;20(22):4453–8.

97. Anderson GS, Brinkmann F, Soulen MC, et al. FDG positron emission tomography in the surveillance of hepatic tumors treated with radiofrequency ablation. Clin Nucl Med 2003;28(3):192–7.

98. Donckier V, Van Laethem JL, Goldman S, et al. [F-18] fluorodeoxyglucose positron emission tomography as a tool for early recognition of incomplete tumor destruction after radiofrequency ablation for liver metastases. J Surg Oncol 2003;84(4):215–23.

99. Blokhuis TJ, van der Schaaf MC, van den Tol MP, et al. Results of radio frequency ablation of primary and secondary liver tumors: long-term follow-up with computed tomography and positron emission tomography-18F-deoxyfluoroglucose scanning. Scand J Gastroenterol Suppl 2004;241:93–7.

100. Barker DW, Zagoria RJ, Morton KA, et al. Evaluation of liver metastases after radiofrequency ablation: utility of 18F-FDG PET and PET/CT. AJR Am J Roentgenol 2005;184(4):1096–102.

101. Joosten J, Jager G, Oyen W, et al. Cryosurgery and radiofrequency ablation for unresectable colorectal liver metastases. Eur J Surg Oncol 2005;31(10): 1152–9.

102. Amthauer H, Denecke T, Hildebrandt B, et al. Evaluation of patients with liver metastases from colorectal cancer for locally ablative treatment with laser induced thermotherapy. Impact of PET with 18F-fluorodeoxyglucose on therapeutic decisions. Nuklearmedizin 2006;45(4):177–84.

103. Denecke T, Steffen I, Hildebrandt B, et al. Assessment of local control after laser-induced thermotherapy of liver metastases from colorectal cancer: contribution of FDG-PET in patients with clinical suspicion of progressive disease. Acta Radiol 2007;48(8):821–30.

104. Khandani AH, Calvo BF, O'Neil BH, et al. A pilot study of early 18F-FDG PET to evaluate the effectiveness of radiofrequency ablation of liver metastases. AJR Am J Roentgenol 2007;189(5): 1199–202.

105. Kuehl H, Antoch G, Stergar H, et al. Comparison of FDG-PET, PET/CT and MRI for follow-up of colorectal liver metastases treated with radiofrequency ablation: initial results. Eur J Radiol 2008;67(2): 362–71.

106. Travaini LL, Trifiro G, Ravasi L, et al. Role of [18F] FDG-PET/CT after radiofrequency ablation of liver metastases: preliminary results. Eur J Nucl Med Mol Imaging 2008;35(7):1316–22.

107. Dierckx R, Maes A, Peeters M, et al. FDG PET for monitoring response to local and locoregional therapy in HCC and liver metastases. Q J Nucl Med Mol Imaging 2009;53(3):336–42.

108. Han AR, Gwak GY, Choi MS, et al. The clinical value of 18F-FDG PET/CT for investigating unexplained serum AFP elevation following interventional therapy for hepatocellular carcinoma. Hepatogastroenterology 2009;56(93):1111–6.

109. Higashi T, Hatano E, Ikai I, et al. FDG PET as a prognostic predictor in the early post-therapeutic evaluation for unresectable hepatocellular carcinoma. Eur J Nucl Med Mol Imaging 2010;37(3): 468–82.

110. Sahin DA, Agcaoglu O, Chretien C, et al. The utility of PET/CT in the management of patients with colorectal liver metastases undergoing laparoscopic radiofrequency thermal ablation. Ann Surg Oncol 2012;19(3):850–5.

111. Chen W, Zhuang H, Cheng G, et al. Comparison of FDG-PET, MRI and CT for post radiofrequency ablation evaluation of hepatic tumors. Ann Nucl Med 2013;27(1):58–64.

112. Nielsen K, van Tilborg AA, Meijerink MR, et al. Incidence and treatment of local site recurrences following RFA of colorectal liver metastases. World J Surg 2013;37(6):1340–7.

113. Wang XY, Chen D, Zhang XS, et al. Value of (1)(8)
     F-FDG-PET/CT in the detection of recurrent hepato-
     cellular carcinoma after hepatectomy or radiofre-
     quency ablation: a comparative study with
     contrast-enhanced ultrasound. J Dig Dis 2013;
     14(8):433–8.

114. Kornberg A, Witt U, Matevossian E, et al. Extended
     postinterventional tumor necrosis-implication for
     outcome in liver transplant patients with advanced
     HCC. PLoS One 2013;8(1):e53960.

115. Vandenbroucke F, Vandemeulebroucke J, Ilsen B,
     et al. Predictive value of pattern classification 24
     hours after radiofrequency ablation of liver metas-
     tases on CT and positron emission tomography/
     CT. J Vasc Interv Radiol 2014;25(8):1240–9.

116. Zheng JH, Chang ZH, Han CB, et al. Detection of
     residual tumor following radiofrequency ablation
     of liver metastases using 18F-FDG PET/PET-CT: a
     systematic review and meta-analysis. Nucl Med
     Commun 2014;35(4):339–46.

Utility of PET for Radiotherapy Treatment Planning

Beant S. Gill, MD[a], Sarah S. Pai, MD[b],
Stacey McKenzie, CNMT, RT (N), (CT)[a], Sushil Beriwal, MD[a],*

KEYWORDS

- PET • Radiation therapy • Radiotherapy • Simulation • Cancer

KEY POINTS

- PET imaging allows for improved oncologic staging and can aid in target delineation for radiotherapy.
- Considerable work has been completed to demonstrate the value of PET/CT for radiotherapy planning, showing that in several disease sites, this approach can lead to more accurate tumor targeting and can alter radiotherapy plans significantly.
- Continued studies are needed to better establish consistent contouring protocols using PET imaging to decrease contoured volume variability.

Advances in diagnostic imaging have led to tremendous clinical implications by altering patient management via improved clinical staging and aiding in targeted treatment. Within the realm of clinical oncology, the discovery and application of PET is largely credited for such advancement. In radiation oncology, where accuracy and precision are paramount, integration of PET with computed tomography (CT) and/or MR imaging has aided in treatment planning, appropriate patient selection, and prognostication in follow-up. Here, we review the techniques of PET imaging in the context of radiation therapy planning and discuss clinical implications in various disease subsites.

OVERVIEW OF ^{18}F-2-FLUORO-2-DEOXY-D-GLUCOSE PET

The crux of PET imaging arises from injection of a radiolabeled molecule into a patient's bloodstream, such that selective uptake by tissue enables more specific imaging. At present, most PET imaging for oncology patients uses ^{18}F-2-fluoro-2-deoxy-D-glucose (^{18}F-FDG). PET using ^{18}F-FDG capitalizes on metabolically active tissues, which preferentially take up glucose at a higher rate than other tissues and thus take up this glucose analog. The addition of a 2′ hydroxyl group inhibits cellular glycolysis, and phosphorylation of the internalized molecule prevents cellular release. In essence, the FDG molecule remains trapped within the cell, unable to undergo further metabolism. The half-life of ^{18}F is 109.8 minutes. Resultant decay of this radioisotope leads to β^+ decay, also known as positron emission. Annihilation of the emitted positron occurs when combined with a nearby electron, resulting in 2 gamma photons moving in opposite directions that are detected by the imager. Thus, metabolic tissues with preferential uptake of ^{18}F-FDG are imaged. As radioactive decay occurs,

The authors have nothing to disclose.
[a] Department of Radiation Oncology, University of Pittsburgh Cancer Institute, 5230 Centre Avenue, Pittsburgh, PA 15232, USA; [b] Department of Radiology, University of Pittsburgh Medical Center, 200 Lothrop Street, Pittsburgh, PA 15213, USA
* Corresponding author. Department of Radiation Oncology, University of Pittsburgh Medical Center, Magee-Womens Hospital, 300 Halket Street, Pittsburgh, PA 15213.
E-mail address: beriwals@upmc.edu

PET Clin 10 (2015) 541–554
http://dx.doi.org/10.1016/j.cpet.2015.05.002
1556-8598/15/$ – see front matter © 2015 Elsevier Inc. All rights reserved.

the molecule converts to glucose-6-phosphate with an attached 2' hydroxyl, allowing for normal metabolism.

Although most tumor cells are generally metabolically active and therefore take up FDG, other physiologically active tissues, such as bowel, cardiac muscle, and brain parenchyma can contribute to normal signal detected on PET. Furthermore, because the by-products of ^{18}F-FDG are renally excreted, concentration in the kidneys, ureters, and bladder can lead to normal uptake. Other non–cancer-specific uptake can occur with tissues involved in an inflammatory or infectious process. For these reasons, careful diagnostic assessment and incorporation of alternative imaging modalities, such as CT or MR imaging, can aid in avoiding false-positive readings.

PET/COMPUTED TOMOGRAPHY SIMULATION TECHNIQUE

Although PET images can be fused to radiotherapy planning imaging, ideally both sets of imaging are completed simultaneously to prevent common errors with image fusion. We discuss here the technique used to complete PET/CT simulation for radiotherapy planning, which is based on our institutional protocol. Other institutional approaches can be found elsewhere.

Radiotherapy simulation involves acquisition of images to allow for accurate and precise treatment planning. Anatomic information can be used not only to guide targeting of at-risk or cancerous regions, but also normal structures that may be avoided. In the modern era, 3-dimensional imaging is often completed using CT, MR imaging, and/or ultrasound. PET/CT is commonly used at our institution for most malignancies. Indications for PET/CT in radiotherapy treatment planning are discussed in the next section.

Patients are instructed to fast 4 to 6 hours before their appointment, with additional restrictions regarding medications taken. Before injection, blood glucose levels are checked to prevent abnormal variability in glucose uptake. A water-soluble iodinated oral contrast is given if identification of the gastrointestinal tract is necessary. Intravenous injection of ^{18}F-FDG is then completed with weight-based dosing (typically 12–20 mCi). After injection, patients remain in a dark, quiet room for approximately 60 minutes. Unless treatment planning with a full bladder is indicated, patients then void before scanning.

At our institution, patients are positioned on a GE Discovery ST (GE Healthcare, Buckinghamshire, UK) scanner. Immobilization approaches vary based on the target region: wingboard for thorax and abdomen, thermoplastic mask for head/neck, arms down for pelvis. All imaging is completed in the same patient position. Imaging typically involves a low-dose CT or diagnostic/high-resolution CT followed by PET image acquisition, the former for attenuation correction. For gynecologic patients, both full and empty bladder CT scanning is completed. Intravenous iodine-based contrast is used for the CT portion if indicated. PET acquisition occurs at 3.27-mm slices, whereas CT slice thickness varies based on radiotherapy modality. For nonstereotactic radiotherapy treatments, 2.5-mm slices are obtained, as opposed to 1.25-mm slice thickness for stereotactic radiotherapy planning.

Images are then imported to the treatment planning software. Image fusion to the CT simulation scan occurs through either rigid or deformable registration. By completing a PET scan at the time of simulation, errors in image registration are often decreased. Because of potential differences in patient positioning over the time of completing the PET and CT scans, fused images should be carefully checked, with particular attention to disease-related regions, to avoid misregistration. Window and level parameters can result in significant variations in tumor contouring and thus should be standardized to each scanner. Tumor volumes from anatomic information (via CT or MR imaging) and physiologic data (via PET) can then be delineated to enable accurate target definition.

TREATMENT PLANNING AND CLINICAL IMPLICATIONS
Head and Neck Cancer

Head and neck squamous cell carcinoma (HNSCC) remains a common worldwide malignancy, with approximately half of patients having advanced disease at presentation. Local therapies are often challenged by nearby critical organs and selection of management approach is driven by clinical stage; thus, accurate pretreatment staging is critical.

PET/CT enables more accurate detection of nodal and distant metastases for HNSCC, particularly in scenarios in which the risk of such metastases is high: locally advanced disease and/or primary sites such as nasopharynx, posterior pharyngeal wall, and hypopharynx. A German prospective trial using PET/CT for IVA/B HNSCC identified 57.1% of patients who had alterations in nodal status, 17.1% with previously undiscovered distant metastases, and 11.4% with a new second primary, which this population is often at risk of developing.[1] In a multicenter, prospective French study, 233 patients with HNSCC had treatment decisions based on CT and/or MR imaging and then were rediscussed after PET or PET/CT.[2] Staging discordance was noted in 43% of patients; PET staging sensitivity and specificity were 91% and 63% compared with CT and/or MR imaging staging that yielded 9% sensitivity and 37% specificity. The investigators thus concluded that PET had improved staging accuracy, leading to management changes in 5.2% to 8.6% of patients. A comparable multicenter study found similar results with a slightly higher rate (33.8%) of management alterations due to PET imaging, although this may be because of a larger population of patients with unknown primary tumors, which can drastically change management.[3] In summary, PET staging should be strongly considered for patients with advanced or high-risk HNSCC because of improved nodal staging, detection of metastases, and identification of synchronous secondary malignancies.

For head and neck cancer of unknown primary (HNC-UP), PET/CT can provide added value for primary site detection. Among studies using PET/CT for HNC-UP, sites of the primary tumor were identified in 29% to 55% of patients.[4–10] Diagnostic yield can be higher when added to additional imaging, endoscopy under anesthesia, and pan-biopsies. Yet, false-positive rates can reach 50% along recently biopsied areas and PET often underassesses mucosal areas, leading to widely variable negative predictive values (25%–96%).[4–10] For these reasons, PET/CT should not be a substitute but rather an adjunct to pan-endoscopy and biopsies. Nonetheless, identification of the primary site can drive management

and may lead to smaller radiotherapy fields, avoiding added toxicity to uninvolved organs.

Our institution conducted an early experience of integrating PET with radiotherapy planning for HNSCC.[11] With 21 cases, PET identified the gross tumor volume (GTV) in all cases and additional sites of disease in 8 cases, whereas the GTV was unidentifiable by CT in 3 cases. Several other studies have confirmed the utility of PET-based radiotherapy planning for HNSCC, showing smaller GTVs when using PET as compared with CT alone.[12–16] Smaller GTV can translate into less normal tissue being irradiated and subsequently less toxicity. However, whether contoured GTVs are truly representative of disease has been less established. Murphy and colleagues[17] reported on 23 patients with oral tongue SCC who had PET/CT before surgery; although metabolic tumor volume was associated with pathologic volume, the strength of the correlation was poor. Yet, compared with CT and MR imaging, PET imaging correlates best with pathologic volume, even though all methods overestimated GTVs.[16,18] Because of variability in pathologic correlation and the devastating impact of locoregional recurrence for HNSCC, our institution incorporates PET/CT for treatment planning as an additive tool rather than as an exclusive method to determine the GTV.

Regarding nodal contouring, PET/CT can often identify nodal metastases not seen on other modalities, as discussed previously. Such findings can lead to modifications in radiotherapy fields (Table 1).[1] Presumably, this benefit would be

Table 1
Studies evaluating the impact of PET imaging on alterations in management and/or radiotherapy treatment plans

Study	n	Treatment Site	Imaging Modality	Change in Management Approach, %	Change in Radiotherapy Plan, %
Schwartz et al,[18] 2005	36	Head and Neck	PET/CT	25.0	13.9
Dietl et al,[1] 2008	35	Head and Neck	PET/CT	17.1	57.1
Subedi et al,[36] 2009	161	Lung	PET/CT	41.0	—
MacManus et al,[37] 2001	153	Lung	PET	30.1	27.0
De Ruysscher et al,[46] 2005	21	Lung	PET/CT	—	66.7
Bradley et al,[40] 2012	52	Lung	PET/CT	3.8	51.1
Leong et al,[63] 2006	21	Esophagus	PET/CT	23.8	68.8
Nguyen et al,[74] 2008	50	Anus	PET or PET/CT	4.0	18.8
Winton et al,[75] 2009	61	Anus	PET or PET/CT	16.4	13.1
Bannas et al,[76] 2011	22	Anus	PET/CT	—	22.7
Krengli et al,[77] 2010	27	Anus	PET/CT	7.4	55.6
Kruser et al,[88] 2009	15	Cervix	PET/CT	26.7	86.7

maximized in patients with otherwise suspected node-negative disease; however, data thus far suggest PET has substantially lower sensitivity in this scenario. Using preoperative imaging for oral cavity SCC, PET resulted in only 70% sensitivity for clinically node-negative disease.[19] The presence of small nodal metastases may account for this difference, mirrored by findings of pathologic node-negative disease in 67% despite being clinically node-negative.[20] Overall, integration of PET/CT for radiotherapy planning can aid in identification of the primary site, result in smaller GTVs, and guide nodal treatment volumes. Limitations of PET integration include underassessment of mucosal disease, false-positive uptake (such as after biopsy, inflammation, or infection), and limited utility in the clinically node-negative neck.

Moving forward, investigators have begun to evaluate PET-directed dose escalation. A phase I trial from Belgium reported feasibility delivering a simultaneous integrated boost to the PET-defined GTV and showing a 1-year local control of 85% to 87%.[21] Additional trials are needed before this approach is routinely adopted, particularly in light of considerable contouring variability without a standardized contouring protocol (**Fig. 1**).[22]

Lung: Non–Small Cell Lung Cancer

PET/CT has become a standard imaging modality for initial staging in non–small cell lung cancer (NSCLC), as recommended by National Comprehensive Cancer Network (NCCN) guidelines.[23] The predominant advantage arises from improved detection of regional and distant metastases. In a meta-analysis of 19 studies, CT staging resulted in mediastinal lymph node metastasis sensitivity and specificity of 55% and 81%, whereas PET staging led to sensitivity and specificity of 77% and 86%.[24] Combined information from PET/CT can further decrease false-negative rates, particularly with presence of nodal enlargement and FDG avidity.[25,26] Nonetheless, mediastinal surgical staging remains the gold standard due to palpable false-negative rates with PET/CT (5%–10%), particularly when lymph nodes are smaller than 7 to 10 mm.[27]

Similar to findings regarding mediastinal staging, PET/CT has led to greater detection of distant metastases. Although the incidence of radiographic metastases varies by stage, among patients with advanced NSCLC, PET imaging identified unsuspected metastatic disease in 6% to 37% of cases.[28–32] As a result, PET staging has led to stage migration, evidenced by population-based analyses. In the Surveillance,

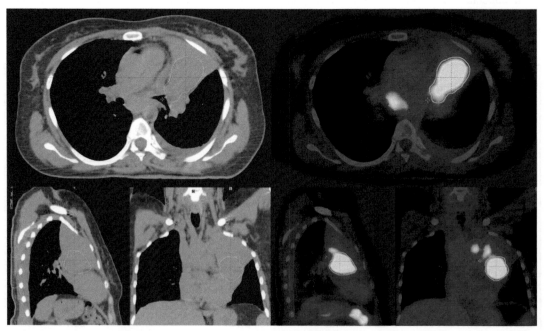

Fig. 1. Gross tumor volume (*light blue*) for a locally advanced NSCLC. PET/CT (*right*), acquired for radiotherapy simulation, identifies the primary tumor based on FDG avidity, whereas CT (*left*) fails to delineate tumor from adjacent right lower lobe atelectasis.

Epidemiology, and End Results (SEER) registry, between 1998 and 2003, PET adoption increased from 2% to 47% among patients with NSCLC, leading to a 5.1% absolute increase in patients with stage IV disease.[33]

Improved staging, such as that seen with PET imaging, has resulted in clinical improvements by decreasing the number of noncurative thoracotomy by approximately one-half.[34,35] Retrospective series identified 21.3% to 30.0% of patients who had changes to management based on PET imaging.[36,37] Although several studies have identified improvements in survival with PET staging, a confounding point is the presence of stage migration and selection bias as a result.[33,38] Still, integration of PET/CT staging can have additional impact on local therapies, guiding targeting through radiotherapy planning.

Target delineation for lung cancer can be particularly challenging given adjacent or overlapping densities and respiratory motion. In cases in which atelectasis or consolidation is present, obscuring clear demarcation of the primary tumor, the addition of PET imaging can be particularly advantageous (**Fig. 2**).[39,40] To account for respiratory motion, our institution uses 4-dimensional (4D) PET/CT, which accounts for respiratory motion at the time of simulation with both CT and PET image acquisition. Initial data using 4D-PET/CT resulted in increases in the maximum standardized uptake value (SUV_{max}) and confirmation of tumor motion assessed by 4D-CT.[41,42] Aristophanous and colleagues[43] reported on radiotherapy treatment planning using 10 patients with NSCLC undergoing both 3D-PET/CT and 4D-PET/CT scans. Despite using 3 different methods of PET-based contouring, 3D-PET/CT volumes were routinely smaller (mean 16%–63%) than 4D-PET/CT volumes, highlighting tumor motion that is otherwise uncaptured on 3D-PET/CT.

Even for facilities without 4D-PET/CT capabilities, PET fusion provides the added benefit of better identifying involved nodal disease. Elective nodal irradiation for NSCLC has fallen out of favor based on data confirming a low incidence of out-of-field isolated nodal recurrences.[44,45] Use of involved nodal irradiation also led to lower rates of pneumonitis and subsequently improved survival.[45] Applying this same concept, PET imaging can lead to more accurate definition of nodal volumes through its improved detection of nodal involvement. In a prospective study from the Netherlands, PET/CT simulation led to radiotherapy field changes in 14 of 21 cases.[46] In turn, esophageal and lung dosimetric parameters were improved; for example, the mean lung dose decreased from 15.6 Gy to 10.5 Gy (*P*<.001). A similar trial conducted in North America, Radiation

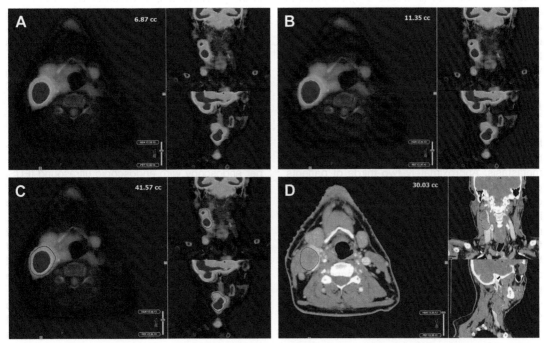

Fig. 2. Challenges with SUV threshold cutoffs in an oropharyngeal cancer with involved cervical neck nodes. Using SUV thresholds of 50% (*A*), 40% (*B*), and 20% (*C*) results in considerable volumetric differences in contoured tumor (area encircled by *red line*) around an involved cervical neck node compared with a CT-defined volume (*D*).

Therapy Oncology Group (RTOG) 0515, confirmed modification of nodal contours in 51% of patients when using PET/CT compared with CT alone.[40] Again, GTVs were reduced (86.2 cm^3 vs 98.7 cm^3, P<.0001), leading to a trend in reduction of mean lung dose (17.8 vs 19.0 Gy, P = .06). Thus, integration of PET for treatment planning of NSCLC has clear implications by reducing treatment volumes, ensuring accurate coverage of involved nodal regions, and, when fields are altered, reducing normal lung dose.

Following radiotherapy, PET response based on SUV$_{max}$ has been correlated with clinical prognosis.[47,48] In a prospective study with 73 patients, PET response remained the only significant predictor for survival on multivariate analysis.[47] American College of Radiology Imaging Network (ACRIN) 6668/RTOG 0235 corroborated these findings following chemoradiation, showing 3-month posttreatment SUV$_{peak}$ and SUV$_{max}$ predicted for survival.[48] Assessment of treatment response based on a single PET/CT after radiotherapy should be taken cautiously though, because of inflammatory posttreatment changes.[49] To allow for alteration in treatment for nonresponders, interval PET/CT during treatment is presently being evaluated. In single-institutional experiences, midtreatment PET/CT has been shown to correlate with posttreatment response and survival.[50,51] The ongoing phase II trial RTOG 1106/ACRIN 6697 incorporates midtreatment PET/CT (in weeks 3–4). All patients undergo carboplatin/paclitaxel chemoradiation, although patients randomized to arm 2 have resimulation and adaptive radiotherapy based on PET/CT response, allowing for dose escalation via hypofractionation.

Lung: Small Cell Lung Cancer

Small cell lung cancer (SCLC) is an aggressive, less common variant of lung cancers with a high propensity for disease recurrence and distant metastasis. Approximately two-thirds of patients present with extensive stage (ES-SCLC) disease on presentation, defined as disease beyond 1 hemithorax or that cannot be confined to a single radiotherapy portal.[52] Applying a similar rationale for upfront staging as that seen in NSCLC, integration of PET/CT for initial staging can improve detection of nodal and distant metastases for suspected limited-stage SCLC (LS-SCLC). Although supporting data regarding PET staging for LS-SCLC is limited to small, single-institution series, recent modifications to the NCCN guidelines convey changing practice patterns with the recommendation for using PET/CT for suspected LS-SCLC cases.[53–55] In a review of 12 studies

using pretreatment PET for LS-SCLC, 19% of patients were upstaged to ES-SCLC and 11% were downstaged.[55] In 6 of these studies, PET findings altered management in 27% of patients. Xanthopoulos and colleagues[54] evaluated 54 LS-SCLC patients who underwent concurrent chemoradiation, findings that those staged with PET had improved median survival (32 vs 17 months, P = .03), which was upheld on multivariate analysis. These findings likely reflect more accurate staging, which can alter management approach and radiotherapy localization.

Early clinical trials evaluating radiotherapy involved use of elective nodal irradiation, covering hilar, mediastinal, and/or supraclavicular lymph nodes. In many of these trials, pretreatment staging did not consist of advanced imaging techniques, such as CT or PET. For this reason, the impact of elective nodal irradiation was evaluated in 2 separate phase II prospective trials in the Netherlands.[56,57] The first trial used CT for staging, delivering involved field radiotherapy with concurrent carboplatin and etoposide.[56] Isolated nodal failure rates were felt to be unacceptably high (11%). However, in a subsequent trial using PET staging, the addition of PET led to alteration in mediastinal staging in 30% of patients.[57] Notably, 5% of patients had supraclavicular involvement on PET that was otherwise uncaptured by CT, which may have accounted for the isolated nodal failures in the previous trial, of which all occurred in the ipsilateral supraclavicular fossa. With PET staging and PET-guided planning, isolated nodal failures were reduced to 3%. Thus, PET staging allows exclusion of elective nodal regions from radiotherapy, which has been shown to reduce lung and esophageal toxicity in previous NSCLC studies.

Gastrointestinal: Esophageal Cancer

Staging for esophageal cancer typically involves upper endoscopy with endoscopic ultrasound (EUS) for local and nodal disease extent and chest/abdomen CT or PET/CT to assess for metastatic disease. Similar to other malignancies discussed, PET/CT can have added utility in the detection of metastatic disease.[58,59] The American College of Surgeons Oncology Group (ACOSOG) Z0060 trial prospectively staged 262 patients with resectable esophageal cancer who were randomized to standard staging with or without PET imaging. Nine patients (4.8%) had pathologically confirmed PET-only determined metastatic disease, with an additional 18 (9.5%) patients with PET-positive histologically unconfirmed metastases.[59] On the other hand, accuracy of nodal staging has varied in published series.[60,61] In a systematic review, van Westreenen and colleagues[60] reported PET nodal staging yielded 51% sensitivity and 84% specificity, but 67% sensitivity and 97% specificity for distant nodal and metastatic assessment. In a Finnish prospective study, accuracy for nodal metastases was slightly inferior with PET compared with other modalities: 63% with PET, 66% with CT, and 75% with EUS.[61] Such findings may reflect frequent presence of subcentimeter nodal metastases and difficulty in assessing para-esophageal nodes near esophageal tumor or physiologic uptake.

In relation to radiotherapy planning, PET/CT offers better estimation of longitudinal tumor length compared with CT alone.[62] In a prospective study evaluating PET/CT for radiotherapy planning, Leong and colleagues[63] discovered that GTVs contoured by CT alone would have excluded PET-avid disease in 69% of patients, again predominantly related to underassessment of longitudinal extent. Challenges with determining an SUV cutoff for contouring remain, although most studies have suggested an SUV_{max} cutoff of 2.5 allows closest estimation of tumor length.[64–66] Within our institution, PET/CT, when completed, is used as a supplementary tool to guide primary treatment volumes, integrated with information from endoscopy and EUS.

Recent approaches with PET/CT involve assessment of response during the course of treatment. In the MUNICON (Metabolic response evalUatioN for Individualisation of neoadjuvant Chemotherapy in oesOphageal and oesophago-gastric adeNocarcinoma) trial, patients with gastroesophageal junction adenocarcinoma received induction chemotherapy followed by PET/CT, with subsequent alteration in chemotherapy based on imaging response.[67] Using a cutoff of 35% decrease in SUV_{max}, metabolic non-responders had worse survival (hazard ratio 2.18, $P = .002$) and higher rates of pathologic response defined as less than 10% residual tumor (58% vs 0%, $P = .001$). These findings have led to the ongoing Cancer and Leukemia Group B (CALGB) 80803 study, a randomized phase III study using PET/CT response to drive neoadjuvant chemotherapy regimen selection (folinic acid, fluorouracil, oxaliplatin [FOLFOX] vs carboplatin/paclitaxel) with radiotherapy.

Gastrointestinal: Gastric and Rectal Cancer

At present, limited evidence exists to support routine use of PET/CT for gastric or rectal cancer. Brush and colleagues[68] conducted a systematic review of studies using PET/CT for staging of colorectal cancer, demonstrating significant heterogeneity and overall insufficient evidence. Physiologic uptake along the rectum and stomach likely contribute to difficulty in adequate assessment of local extent of disease. Furthermore, because metastases frequently occur within the liver, identification of metastases is often better assessed by MR imaging.[69] Guidelines from the European Organisation for Research and Treatment of Cancer have thus recommended against PET/CT for gastric cancer.[70]

Gastrointestinal: Anal Cancer

The role of PET/CT for anal cancer staging continues to evolve, particularly given that only 48.5% of patients present with localized disease.[71] Patients with anal squamous cell carcinoma are generally managed with chemoradiation, given high rates of disease control, allowing for sphincter preservation.[72] Although MR imaging provides superior soft tissue differentiation, staging PET/CT allows accurate assessment of nodal and distant metastases.[72,73] In a systematic review, Caldarella and colleagues[73] identified that PET-based nodal staging yielded a pooled sensitivity and specificity of 56% and 90%, respectively. Although specificity remains high when nodes are FDG-avid, the low sensitivity remains a concern, which may reflect the propensity of having multiple, subcentimeter nodal metastases below PET detection thresholds.

Given the high risk of nodal metastases in anal cancer, for most patients, radiotherapy is directed to the inguinal and pelvic lymph nodes regardless of involvement. Thus, changes based on PET/CT findings would be related to prescribed total dose as opposed to initial radiotherapy fields.[74–76] Nguyen and colleagues[74] identified 19% of patients in whom staging PET/CT resulted in changes to radiotherapy planning, mainly related to dose to those regions. When using PET/CT for radiotherapy simulation, Krengli and colleagues[77] noted GTV contour changes in 55.6% of patients, resulting in smaller GTVs compared with CT-based GTVs. Although dose alterations and smaller GTVs leading to smaller high-dose fields may theoretically improve radiotherapy planning, whether such changes will lead to less toxicity or fewer recurrences remains unknown for anal cancer. Because of the low sensitivity of PET in this setting, radiation oncologists should be cautious in excluding or prescribing suboptimal doses to inguinal nodes based on PET findings.

Gynecologic: Cervical Cancer

Patients with cervical cancer with bulky, node-positive, and/or locally advanced disease typically receive definitive chemoradiation, whereas remaining patients with nonmetastatic disease undergo upfront surgery. Therefore, although International Federation of Gynecology and Obstetrics (FIGO) staging does not incorporate radiographic findings, nodal staging can have a tremendous impact on clinical management. In a prospective cohort study using PET or PET/CT staging for patients with cervical cancer, Kidd and colleagues[78] identified 47% with PET-positive nodal disease. The incidence of PET-based nodal involvement based on stage appeared comparable to historical surgical series. PET-based nodal status correlated with recurrence-free and disease-specific survival. Reliable detection of nodal disease though often relies on FIGO stage; pelvic nodal sensitivity and specificity with PET is 53 to 72 and 90.0% to 99.7% for FIGO stage IA-IIA disease, compared with 75.0% and 96.0% for more advanced disease.[79–81] PET imaging still remains superior for nodal staging compared with CT or MR imaging alone, with even higher sensitivity using combined PET/CT.[82–84] For these reasons, our institution typically uses PET/CT for staging in all patients with locally advanced cervical cancer (FIGO stage IB2 or greater).

Although sensitivity appears high for pelvic nodal assessment, controversy exists regarding utility for para-aortic staging. Overall, sensitivity of PET staging for para-aortic nodes appears low at 34%, as shown in a meta-analysis.[85] However, among high-risk patients (prevalence of para-aortic nodal metastases >15%), pooled sensitivity improved to 73%, likely reflective of a higher incidence of macroscopic metastases rather than microscopic, subcentimeter nodal metastases. Similarly, presence of pelvic nodal involvement can alter the risk of false-positive rates for para-aortic nodal involvement. In 2 prospective trials, the false-negative rate for para-aortic involvement was 8% to 12% for patients without PET-positive nodal disease, which increased to 18% to 22% with PET-positive pelvic lymph nodes.[86,87] For this reason, PET findings can drive nodal radiotherapy volumes. Extended field radiotherapy (EFRT) is used prophylactically to cover the para-aortic lymph nodes. Although no consensus exists regarding when to use EFRT, we typically recommend EFRT for patients with pelvic node–positive disease given the high false-negative rate for para-aortic nodal involvement (**Fig. 3**).

Incorporation of PET/CT for radiotherapy planning to define the primary tumor extent appears less well established. Kruser and colleagues[88] conducted a prospective study using PET/CT simulation, where among patients with cervical cancer, 60% (9 of 15) had changes to GTV greater than 20%. Conversely, MR imaging is a competing modality with superior definition of local tumor compared with CT.[89] In a comparative study between PET/CT and MR imaging, MR imaging and PET/CT GTVs were similar for smaller tumors, although MR imaging was a superior method for

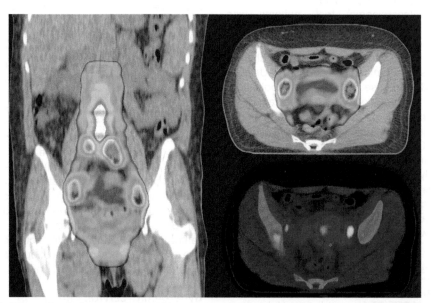

Fig. 3. Radiotherapy simulation PET/CT identifying FDG-avid bilateral distal common and external iliac lymphadenopathy (*bottom right*) in a patient with stage IIIB cervical cancer. Dose color wash (*top right* and *left*) is shown to highlight the prescription isodose line on the radiotherapy treatment plan, which was altered to deliver a simultaneous integrated boost to involved lymph nodes as well as prophylactic coverage of para-aortic nodes.

bulkier tumors.[90] Targeting of metabolically active disease has been piloted with the Washington University of St Louis group, using a metabolic threshold of 40% of the SUV_{max} to delineate the GTV.[91,92] Overall, local control rates appear favorable; how much of this improvement compared with historical data is a result of FDG-driven contouring is unclear. PET/MR appears to have growing utility, acquiring benefits of each imaging modality, which may allow for improved radiotherapy target delineation.[93] Establishing appropriate PET/MR thresholds for contouring is already under way.[94]

Challenges and Pitfalls

Although PET/CT for radiotherapy planning has clear utility in some disease sites, there are a number of challenges that remain. Contouring protocols vary tremendously, which can have a substantial impact on tumor volumes.[22,95,96] At present, various techniques exist for segmentation of target volumes from PET imaging: manual contouring, thresholding, and gradient edge detection. Manual contouring consists of physician determination of the tumor outline based on visual inspection. Thresholding uses a minimum SUV value to identify the target.[97] Gradient edge detection delineates tumor based on the changes in signal across a given area.[98,99] Normalization methods can additionally result in contouring variations; at our institution and others, values are typically normalized relative to background liver activity.[11,100]

Initial investigative approaches were focused on SUV thresholding. For NSCLC, optimal SUV thresholds vary from 31% to 50% using pathologic or CT correlation.[101–103] Alternatively, source-to-background ratios have been used for contouring, correlating with gross specimens and reducing interobserver variability.[96,104] For head and neck cancers, varying thresholds have been reported, with data by Burri and colleagues[105] suggesting the most accurate pathologic correlation using a 40% SUV threshold. Our institutional study for recurrent HNSCC demonstrated unacceptable variability using purely automated thresholding techniques.[106] Additionally, small variations in threshold cutoffs can lead to dramatic alterations in volume; Ford and colleagues[95] demonstrated, in some cases, a twofold increase in tumor volume when changing threshold cutoffs by 5% (see **Fig. 2**). Given inconsistencies with threshold methods, alternative segmentation approaches have been investigated. When comparing various contouring methods using a spherical phantom, Werner-Wasik et al.[98] identified gradient edge detection as the most reliable; the mean absolute percentage errors in volume using manual, threshold, and gradient edge methods were 19.5%, 17.5% and 11.0%. Superiority of gradient-based over threshold-based methods has been confirmed in an NSCLC surgical series.[99] At present, further investigation is warranted to determine the clinical impact of gradient edge detection for radiotherapy planning and the optimal autosegmentation approach before widespread adoption.

Additional technical issues regarding target delineation include regions with significant motion and areas with considerable background FDG uptake. The applicability of PET/CT for contouring in brain and gastric malignancies, for example, are challenged by background physiologic uptake. Identification of alternative tumor markers may aid in future applications. Target motion can thus result in PET image blurring, due to the time length of image acquisition, as well as decreases in maximum activity concentration.[107] Implementation of gated 4D-PET/CT, which is used at our institution, can avoid this issue.[43]

SUMMARY

Development and accessibility of PET/CT has considerably changed patient management in oncology, allowing for more accurate clinical staging and target delineation for radiotherapy. Integration with radiotherapy planning, either at the time of simulation or with image fusion, has enabled adaptive planning and has become an additive tool to ensure accurate target delineation. Continued research is needed to establish uniform contouring guidelines and evaluate the clinical impact of PET-based planning, both with regard to toxicity and disease control.

REFERENCES

1. Dietl B, Marienhagen J, Kuhnel T, et al. The impact of FDG-PET/CT on the management of head and neck tumours: the radiotherapist's perspective. Oral Oncol 2008;44(5):504–8.
2. Lonneux M, Hamoir M, Reychler H, et al. Positron emission tomography with [18F]fluorodeoxyglucose improves staging and patient management in patients with head and neck squamous cell carcinoma: a multicenter prospective study. J Clin Oncol 2010;28(7):1190–5.
3. Scott AM, Gunawardana DH, Bartholomeusz D, et al. PET changes management and improves prognostic stratification in patients with head and neck cancer: results of a multicenter prospective study. J Nucl Med 2008;49(10):1593–600.
4. Miller FR, Hussey D, Beeram M, et al. Positron emission tomography in the management of

unknown primary head and neck carcinoma. Arch Otolaryngol Head Neck Surg 2005;131(7):626–9.

5. Rudmik L, Lau HY, Matthews TW, et al. Clinical utility of PET/CT in the evaluation of head and neck squamous cell carcinoma with an unknown primary: a prospective clinical trial. Head Neck 2011;33(7):935–40.

6. Yabuki K, Tsukuda M, Horiuchi C, et al. Role of 18F-FDG PET in detecting primary site in the patient with primary unknown carcinoma. Eur Arch Otorhinolaryngol 2010;267(11):1785–92.

7. Dandekar MR, Kannan S, Rangarajan V, et al. Utility of PET in unknown primary with cervical metastasis: a retrospective study. Indian J Cancer 2011;48(2):181–6.

8. Padovani D, Aimoni C, Zucchetta P, et al. 18-FDG PET in the diagnosis of laterocervical metastases from occult carcinoma. Eur Arch Otorhinolaryngol 2009;266(2):267–71.

9. Johansen J, Buus S, Loft A, et al. Prospective study of 18FDG-PET in the detection and management of patients with lymph node metastases to the neck from an unknown primary tumor. Results from the DAHANCA-13 study. Head Neck 2008;30(4):471–8.

10. Wong WL, Sonoda LI, Gharpurhy A, et al. 18F-fluorodeoxyglucose positron emission tomography/computed tomography in the assessment of occult primary head and neck cancers–an audit and review of published studies. Clin Oncol (R Coll Radiol) 2012;24(3):190–5.

11. Heron DE, Andrade RS, Flickinger J, et al. Hybrid PET-CT simulation for radiation treatment planning in head-and-neck cancers: a brief technical report. Int J Radiat Oncol Biol Phys 2004;60(5):1419–24.

12. Delouya G, Igidbashian L, Houle A, et al. 18F-FDG-PET imaging in radiotherapy tumor volume delineation in treatment of head and neck cancer. Radiother Oncol 2011;101(3):362–8.

13. Paulino AC, Koshy M, Howell R, et al. Comparison of CT- and FDG-PET-defined gross tumor volume in intensity-modulated radiotherapy for head-and-neck cancer. Int J Radiat Oncol Biol Phys 2005; 61(5):1385–92.

14. Guido A, Fuccio L, Rombi B, et al. Combined 18F-FDG-PET/CT imaging in radiotherapy target delineation for head-and-neck cancer. Int J Radiat Oncol Biol Phys 2009;73(3):759–63.

15. Henriques de figueiredo B, Barret O, Demeaux H, et al. Comparison between CT- and FDG-PET-defined target volumes for radiotherapy planning in head-and-neck cancers. Radiother Oncol 2009; 93(3):479–82.

16. Daisne JF, Duprez T, Weynand B, et al. Tumor volume in pharyngolaryngeal squamous cell carcinoma: comparison at CT, MR imaging, and FDG PET and validation with surgical specimen. Radiology 2004;233(1):93–100.

17. Murphy JD, Chisholm KM, Daly ME, et al. Correlation between metabolic tumor volume and pathologic tumor volume in squamous cell carcinoma of the oral cavity. Radiother Oncol 2011;101(3): 356–61.

18. Schwartz DL, Ford E, Rajendran J, et al. FDG-PET/CT imaging for preradiotherapy staging of head-and-neck squamous cell carcinoma. Int J Radiat Oncol Biol Phys 2005;61(1):129–36.

19. Stuckensen T, Kovács AF, Adams S, et al. Staging of the neck in patients with oral cavity squamous cell carcinomas: a prospective comparison of PET, ultrasound, CT and MRI. J Craniomaxillofac Surg 2000;28(6):319–24.

20. Shah JP. Patterns of cervical lymph node metastasis from squamous carcinomas of the upper aerodigestive tract. Am J Surg 1990;160(4):405–9.

21. Madani I, Duthoy W, Derie C, et al. Positron emission tomography-guided, focal-dose escalation using intensity-modulated radiotherapy for head and neck cancer. Int J Radiat Oncol Biol Phys 2007; 68(1):126–35.

22. Riegel AC, Berson AM, Destian S, et al. Variability of gross tumor volume delineation in head-and-neck cancer using CT and PET/CT fusion. Int J Radiat Oncol Biol Phys 2006;65:726–32.

23. National Comprehensive Cancer Network. Non-small cell lung cancer (version 3.2015). Available at: http://www.nccn.org/professionals/physician_gls/pdf/nscl.pdf. Accessed December 15, 2014.

24. Silvestri GA, Gonzalez AV, Jantz MA, et al. Methods for staging non-small cell lung cancer: diagnosis and management of lung cancer, 3rd ed: American College of Chest Physicians evidence-based clinical practice guidelines. Chest 2013;143(5 Suppl): e211S–2150S.

25. Lardinois D, Weder W, Hany TF, et al. Staging of non-small-cell lung cancer with integrated positron-emission tomography and computed tomography. N Engl J Med 2003;348(25):2500–7.

26. Hellwig D, Baum RP, Kirsch C. FDG-PET, PET/CT and conventional nuclear medicine procedures in the evaluation of lung cancer: a systematic review. Nuklearmedizin 2009;48(2):59–69 [quiz: N8–9].

27. Herth FJ, Eberhardt R, Krasnik M, et al. Endobronchial ultrasound-guided transbronchial needle aspiration of lymph nodes in the radiologically and positron emission tomography-normal mediastinum in patients with lung cancer. Chest 2008; 133(4):887–91.

28. Chiba K, Isoda M, Chiba M, et al. Significance of PET/CT in determining actual TNM staging for patients with various lung cancers. Int Surg 2010; 95(3):197–204.

29. Sharma R, Tripathi M, D'souza M, et al. The importance of 18F-FDG PET/CT, CT and X-rays in detecting primary stage III A lung cancer and the

incidence of extra thoracic metastases. Hell J Nucl Med 2009;12(1):22–5.

30. Alonso moralejo R, Sayas catalán J, García luján R, et al. Use of positron emission tomography in assessing hidden extrathoracic metastasis in non small cell lung cancer. Arch Bronconeumol 2010; 46(5):238–43 [in Spanish].

31. MacManus MP, Hicks RJ, Matthews JP, et al. High rate of detection of unsuspected distant metastases by pet in apparent stage III non-small-cell lung cancer: implications for radical radiation therapy. Int J Radiat Oncol Biol Phys 2001; 50(2):287–93.

32. Rodríguez fernández A, Bellón guardia ME, Gómez río M, et al. Staging of non-small cell lung cancer. Diagnosis efficacy of structural (CT) and functional (FDG-PET) imaging methods. Rev Clin Esp 2007; 207(11):541–7 [in Spanish].

33. Dinan MA, Curtis LH, Carpenter WR, et al. Stage migration, selection bias, and survival associated with the adoption of positron emission tomography among Medicare beneficiaries with non-small-cell lung cancer, 1998–2003. J Clin Oncol 2012; 30(22):2725–30.

34. Fischer B, Lassen U, Mortensen J, et al. Preoperative staging of lung cancer with combined PET-CT. N Engl J Med 2009;361(1):32–9.

35. Van Tinteren H, Hoekstra OS, Smit EF, et al. Effectiveness of positron emission tomography in the preoperative assessment of patients with suspected non-small-cell lung cancer: the PLUS multicentre randomised trial. Lancet 2002;359(9315): 1388–93.

36. Subedi N, Scarsbrook A, Darby M, et al. The clinical impact of integrated FDG PET-CT on management decisions in patients with lung cancer. Lung Cancer 2009;64(3):301–7.

37. MacManus MP, Hicks RJ, Ball DL, et al. F-18 fluorodeoxyglucose positron emission tomography staging in radical radiotherapy candidates with nonsmall cell lung carcinoma: powerful correlation with survival and high impact on treatment. Cancer 2001;92(4):886–95.

38. Chee KG, Nguyen DV, Brown M, et al. Positron emission tomography and improved survival in patients with lung cancer: the Will Rogers phenomenon revisited. Arch Intern Med 2008;168(14): 1541–9.

39. Nestle U, Walter K, Schmidt S, et al. 18F-deoxyglucose positron emission tomography (FDG-PET) for the planning of radiotherapy in lung cancer: high impact in patients with atelectasis. Int J Radiat Oncol Biol Phys 1999;44:593–7.

40. Bradley J, Bae K, Choi N, et al. A phase II comparative study of gross tumor volume definition with or without PET/CT fusion in dosimetric planning for non-small-cell lung cancer (NSCLC): primary analysis of Radiation Therapy Oncology Group (RTOG) 0515. Int J Radiat Oncol Biol Phys 2012; 82(1):435–41.e1.

41. Nehmeh SA, Erdi YE, Pan T, et al. Four-dimensional (4D) PET/CT imaging of the thorax. Med Phys 2004;31:3179–86.

42. Wolthaus JW, van Herk M, Muller SH, et al. Fusion of respiratory-correlated PET and CT scans: correlated lung tumour motion in anatomical and functional scans. Phys Med Biol 2005;50:1569–83.

43. Aristophanous M, Berbeco RI, Killoran JH, et al. Clinical utility of 4D FDG-PET/CT scans in radiation treatment planning. Int J Radiat Oncol Biol Phys 2012;82(1):e99–105.

44. Rosenzweig KE, Sura S, Jackson A, et al. Involved-field radiation therapy for inoperable non small-cell lung cancer. J Clin Oncol 2007;25(35):5557–61.

45. Yuan S, Sun X, Li M, et al. A randomized study of involved-field irradiation versus elective nodal irradiation in combination with concurrent chemotherapy for inoperable stage III nonsmall cell lung cancer. Am J Clin Oncol 2007;30(3):239–44.

46. De Ruysscher D, Wanders S, Minken A, et al. Effects of radiotherapy planning with a dedicated combined PET-CT-simulator of patients with non-small cell lung cancer on dose limiting normal tissues and radiation dose-escalation: a planning study. Radiother Oncol 2005;77(1):5–10.

47. MacManus MP, Hicks RJ, Matthews JP, et al. Positron emission tomography is superior to computed tomography scanning for response-assessment after radical radiotherapy or chemoradiotherapy in patients with non-small-cell lung cancer. J Clin Oncol 2003;21(7):1285–92.

48. Machtay M, Duan F, Siegel BA, et al. Prediction of survival by [18F]fluorodeoxyglucose positron emission tomography in patients with locally advanced non-small-cell lung cancer undergoing definitive chemoradiation therapy: results of the ACRIN 6668/RTOG 0235 trial. J Clin Oncol 2013;31(30): 3823–30.

49. Matsuo Y, Nakamoto Y, Nagata Y, et al. Characterization of FDG-PET images after stereotactic body radiation therapy for lung cancer. Radiother Oncol 2010;97(2):200–4.

50. Kong FM, Frey KA, Quint LE, et al. A pilot study of [18F]fluorodeoxyglucose positron emission tomography scans during and after radiation-based therapy in patients with non small-cell lung cancer. J Clin Oncol 2007;25(21):3116–23.

51. Van Elmpt W, Ollers M, Dingemans AM, et al. Response assessment using 18F-FDG PET early in the course of radiotherapy correlates with survival in advanced-stage non-small cell lung cancer. J Nucl Med 2012;53(10):1514–20.

52. Govindan R, Page N, Morgensztern D, et al. Changing epidemiology of small-cell lung cancer

in the United States over the last 30 years: analysis of the surveillance, epidemiologic, and end results database. J Clin Oncol 2006;24(28):4539–44.

53. National Comprehensive Cancer Network. Small cell lung cancer (Version 1.2015). Available at: http://www.nccn.org/professionals/physician_gls/pdf/sclc.pdf. Accessed December 15, 2014.

54. Xanthopoulos EP, Corradetti MN, Mitra N, et al. Impact of PET staging in limited-stage small-cell lung cancer. J Thorac Oncol 2013;8(7):899–905.

55. Kalemkerian GP. Staging and imaging of small cell lung cancer. Cancer Imaging 2011;11:253–8.

56. De Ruysscher D, Bremer RH, Koppe F, et al. Omission of elective node irradiation on basis of CT-scans in patients with limited disease small cell lung cancer: a phase II trial. Radiother Oncol 2006;80(3):307–12.

57. van Loon J, De Ruysscher D, Wanders R, et al. Selective nodal irradiation on basis of (18)FDG-PET scans in limited-disease small-cell lung cancer: a prospective study. Int J Radiat Oncol Biol Phys 2010;77(2):329–36.

58. Flanagan FL, Dehdashti F, Siegel BA, et al. Staging of esophageal cancer with 18F-fluorodeoxyglucose positron emission tomography. AJR Am J Roentgenol 1997;168(2):417–24.

59. Meyers BF, Downey RJ, Decker PA, et al. The utility of positron emission tomography in staging of potentially operable carcinoma of the thoracic esophagus: results of the American College of Surgeons Oncology Group Z0060 trial. J Thorac Cardiovasc Surg 2007;133(3):738–45.

60. van Westreenen HL, Westerterp M, Bossuyt PM, et al. Systematic review of the staging performance of 18F-fluorodeoxyglucose positron emission tomography in esophageal cancer. J Clin Oncol 2004;22(18):3805–12.

61. Räsänen JV, Sihvo EI, Knuuti MJ, et al. Prospective analysis of accuracy of positron emission tomography, computed tomography, and endoscopic ultrasonography in staging of adenocarcinoma of the esophagus and the esophagogastric junction. Ann Surg Oncol 2003;10(8):954–60.

62. Drudi FM, Trippa F, Cascone F, et al. Esophagogram and CT vs endoscopic and surgical specimens in the diagnosis of esophageal carcinoma. Radiol Med 2002;103(4):344–52.

63. Leong T, Everitt C, Yuen K, et al. A prospective study to evaluate the impact of FDG-PET on CT-based radiotherapy treatment planning for oesophageal cancer. Radiother Oncol 2006;78(3):254–61.

64. Zhong X, Yu J, Zhang B, et al. Using 18F-fluorodeoxyglucose positron emission tomography to estimate the length of gross tumor in patients with squamous cell carcinoma of the esophagus. Int J Radiat Oncol Biol Phys 2009;73(1):136–41.

65. Han D, Yu J, Yu Y, et al. Comparison of (18)F-fluorothymidine and (18)F-fluorodeoxyglucose PET/CT in delineating gross tumor volume by optimal threshold in patients with squamous cell carcinoma of thoracic esophagus. Int J Radiat Oncol Biol Phys 2010;76(4):1235–41.

66. Vali FS, Nagda S, Hall W, et al. Comparison of standardized uptake value-based positron emission tomography and computed tomography target volumes in esophageal cancer patients undergoing radiotherapy. Int J Radiat Oncol Biol Phys 2010;78(4):1057–63.

67. Lordick F, Ott K, Krause BJ, et al. PET to assess early metabolic response and to guide treatment of adenocarcinoma of the oesophagogastric junction: the MUNICON phase II trial. Lancet Oncol 2007;8(9):797–805.

68. Brush J, Boyd K, Chappell F, et al. The value of FDG positron emission tomography/computerised tomography (PET/CT) in pre-operative staging of colorectal cancer: a systematic review and economic evaluation. Health Technol Assess 2011;15(35):1–192, iii–iv.

69. Niekel MC, Bipat S, Stoker J. Diagnostic imaging of colorectal liver metastases with CT, MR imaging, FDG PET, and/or FDG PET/CT: a meta-analysis of prospective studies including patients who have not previously undergone treatment. Radiology 2010;257(3):674–84.

70. Lutz MP, Zalcberg JR, Ducreux M, et al. Highlights of the EORTC St. Gallen international expert consensus on the primary therapy of gastric, gastroesophageal and oesophageal cancer—differential treatment strategies for subtypes of early gastroesophageal cancer. Eur J Cancer 2012;48(16):2941–53.

71. Howlander N, Noone AM, Krapcho M, et al. SEER cancer statistics review, 1975–2011. Bethesda (MD): National Cancer Institute; 2014. Based on November 2013 SEER data submission, posted to the SEER Web site. Available at: http://seer.cancer.gov/csr/1975_2011/. Accessed December 18, 2014.

72. Poggi MM, Suh WW, Saltz L, et al. ACR appropriateness criteria on treatment of anal cancer. J Am Coll Radiol 2007;4(7):448–56.

73. Caldarella C, Annunziata S, Treglia G, et al. Diagnostic performance of positron emission tomography/computed tomography using fluorine-18 fluorodeoxyglucose in detecting locoregional nodal involvement in patients with anal canal cancer: a systematic review and meta-analysis. ScientificWorldJournal 2014;2014:196068.

74. Nguyen BT, Joon DL, Khoo V, et al. Assessing the impact of FDG-PET in the management of anal cancer. Radiother Oncol 2008;87(3):376–82.

75. Winton ED, Heriot AG, Ng M, et al. The impact of 18-fluorodeoxyglucose positron emission tomography

on the staging, management and outcome of anal cancer. Br J Cancer 2009;100(5):693–700.

76. Bannas P, Weber C, Adam G, et al. Contrast-enhanced [(18)F]fluorodeoxyglucose-positron emission tomography/computed tomography for staging and radiotherapy planning in patients with anal cancer. Int J Radiat Oncol Biol Phys 2011;81(2):445–51.

77. Krengli M, Milia ME, Turri L, et al. FDG-PET/CT imaging for staging and target volume delineation in conformal radiotherapy of anal carcinoma. Radiat Oncol 2010;5:10.

78. Kidd EA, Siegel BA, Dehdashti F, et al. Lymph node staging by positron emission tomography in cervical cancer: relationship to prognosis. J Clin Oncol 2010;28(12):2108–13.

79. Sironi S, Buda A, Picchio M, et al. Lymph node metastasis in patients with clinical early-stage cervical cancer: detection with integrated FDG PET/CT. Radiology 2006;238(1):272–9.

80. Wright JD, Dehdashti F, Herzog TJ, et al. Preoperative lymph node staging of early-stage cervical carcinoma by [18F]-fluoro-2-deoxy-D-glucose-positron emission tomography. Cancer 2005; 104(11):2484–91.

81. Loft A, Berthelsen AK, Roed H, et al. The diagnostic value of PET/CT scanning in patients with cervical cancer: a prospective study. Gynecol Oncol 2007;106(1):29–34.

82. Reinhardt MJ, Ehritt-Braun C, Vogelgesang D, et al. Metastatic lymph nodes in patients with cervical cancer: detection with MR imaging and FDG PET. Radiology 2001;218(3):776–82.

83. Yen TC, Ng KK, Ma SY, et al. Value of dual-phase 2-fluoro-2-deoxy-d-glucose positron emission tomography in cervical cancer. J Clin Oncol 2003;21(19):3651–8.

84. Metser U, Golan O, Levine CD, et al. Tumor lesion detection: when is integrated positron emission tomography/computed tomography more accurate than side-by-side interpretation of positron emission tomography and computed tomography? J Comput Assist Tomogr 2005;29(4):554–9.

85. Kang S, Kim SK, Chung DC, et al. Diagnostic value of (18)F-FDG PET for evaluation of paraaortic nodal metastasis in patients with cervical carcinoma: a metaanalysis. J Nucl Med 2010;51(3):360–7.

86. Margulies AL, Peres A, Barranger E, et al. Selection of patients with advanced-stage cervical cancer for para-aortic lymphadenectomy in the era of PET/CT. Anticancer Res 2013;33(1):283–6.

87. Ramirez PT, Jhingran A, Macapinlac HA, et al. Laparoscopic extraperitoneal para-aortic lymphadenectomy in locally advanced cervical cancer: a prospective correlation of surgical findings with positron emission tomography/computed tomography findings. Cancer 2011;117(9):1928–34.

88. Kruser TJ, Bradley KA, Bentzen SM, et al. The impact of hybrid PET-CT scan on overall oncologic management, with a focus on radiotherapy planning: a prospective, blinded study. Technol Cancer Res Treat 2009;8(2):149–58.

89. Mitchell DG, Snyder B, Coakley F, et al. Early invasive cervical cancer: tumor delineation by magnetic resonance imaging, computed tomography, and clinical examination, verified by pathologic results, in the ACRIN 6651/GOG 183 Intergroup Study. J Clin Oncol 2006;24(36):5687–94.

90. Ma DJ, Zhu JM, Grigsby PW. Tumor volume discrepancies between FDG-PET and MRI for cervical cancer. Radiother Oncol 2011;98(1):139–42.

91. Kidd EA, Siegel BA, Dehdashti F, et al. Clinical outcomes of definitive intensity-modulated radiation therapy with fluorodeoxyglucose-positron emission tomography simulation in patients with locally advanced cervical cancer. Int J Radiat Oncol Biol Phys 2010;77(4):1085–91.

92. Miller TR, Grigsby PW. Measurement of tumor volume by PET to evaluate prognosis in patients with advanced cervical cancer treated by radiation therapy. Int J Radiat Oncol Biol Phys 2002;53(2):353–9.

93. Kitajima K, Suenaga Y, Ueno Y, et al. Value of fusion of PET and MRI in the detection of intra-pelvic recurrence of gynecological tumor: comparison with 18F-FDG contrast-enhanced PET/CT and pelvic MRI. Ann Nucl Med 2014;28(1):25–32.

94. Zhang S, Xin J, Guo Q, et al. Defining PET tumor volume in cervical cancer with hybrid PET/MRI: a comparative study. Nucl Med Commun 2014; 35(7):712–9.

95. Ford EC, Kinahan PE, Hanlon L, et al. Tumor delineation using PET in head and neck cancers: threshold contouring and lesion volumes. Med Phys 2006;33(11):4280–8.

96. Nestle2 U, Kremp S, Schaefer-Schuler A, et al. Comparison of different methods for delineation of 18F-FDG PET-positive tissue for target volume definition in radiotherapy of patients with non-small cell lung cancer. J Nucl Med 2005;46: 1342–8.

97. Black QC, Grills IS, Kestin LL, et al. Defining a radiotherapy target with positron emission tomography. Int J Radiat Oncol Biol Phys 2004;60(4): 1272–82.

98. Werner-Wasik M, Nelson AD, Choi W, et al. What is the best way to contour lung tumors on PET scans? Multiobserver validation of a gradient-based method using a NSCLC digital PET phantom. Int J Radiat Oncol Biol Phys 2012;82(3):1164–71.

99. Wanet M, Lee JA, Weynand B, et al. Gradient-based delineation of the primary GTV on FDG-PET in non-small cell lung cancer: a comparison with threshold-based approaches, CT and surgical specimens. Radiother Oncol 2011;98(1):117–25.

100. Gondi V, Bradley K, Mehta M, et al. Impact of hybrid fluorodeoxyglucose positron-emission tomography/computed tomography on radiotherapy planning in esophageal and non-small-cell lung cancer. Int J Radiat Oncol Biol Phys 2007;67(1): 187–95.

101. Yu J, Li X, Xing L, et al. Comparison of tumor volumes as determined by pathologic examination and FDG-PET/CT images of non-small-cell lung cancer: a pilot study. Int J Radiat Oncol Biol Phys 2009;75(5):1468–74.

102. Biehl KJ, Kong FM, Dehdashti F, et al. 18F-FDG PET definition of gross tumor volume for radiotherapy of non-small cell lung cancer: is a single standardized uptake value threshold approach appropriate? J Nucl Med 2006;47(11):1808–12.

103. Wu K, Ung YC, Hornby J, et al. PET CT thresholds for radiotherapy target definition in non-small-cell lung cancer: how close are we to the pathologic findings? Int J Radiat Oncol Biol Phys 2010;77(3): 699–706.

104. Van Baardwijk A, Bosmans G, Boersma L, et al. PET-CT-based auto-contouring in non-small-cell lung cancer correlates with pathology and reduces interobserver variability in the delineation of the primary tumor and involved nodal volumes. Int J Radiat Oncol Biol Phys 2007;68(3):771–8.

105. Burri RJ, Rangaswamy B, Kostakoglu L, et al. Correlation of positron emission tomography standard uptake value and pathologic specimen size in cancer of the head and neck. Int J Radiat Oncol Biol Phys 2008;71(3):682–8.

106. Wang K, Heron DE, Clump DA, et al. Target delineation in stereotactic body radiation therapy for recurrent head and neck cancer: a retrospective analysis of the impact of margins and automated PET-CT segmentation. Radiother Oncol 2013; 106(1):90–5.

107. Nehmeh SA, Erdi YE, Ling CC, et al. Effect of respiratory gating on reducing lung motion artifacts in PET imaging of lung cancer. Med Phys 2002; 29(3):366–71.

Applications of Fluorodeoxyglucose PET/Computed Tomography in the Assessment and Prediction of Radiation Therapy–related Complications

Sina Houshmand, MD[a], Ben Boursi, MD[b], Ali Salavati, MD, MPH[a,c],
Charles B. Simone II, MD[d], Abass Alavi, MD[a,*]

KEYWORDS

- Fluorodeoxyglucose PET/Computed tomography • Cancer • Radiation therapy • Complications

KEY POINTS

- Normal tissues respond to radiation therapy in 2 time frames: early or acute effect, which occur days and weeks after irradiation; and late effects, happening months or years after irradiation.
- Radiation pneumonitis is a life-threatening acute and subacute complication of radiation therapy happening in 4% to 30% of patients and manifesting 1 to 6 months after radiation.
- Cardiovascular sequelae are causes of mortality and morbidity related to radiation therapy, and are most well characterized as developing 10 to 15 years after radiation therapy but may be an important cause of treatment-related complications in the months after radiotherapy completion.

INTRODUCTION

Radiation therapy (RT) has an important role in the treatment of many cancer types. The physician's goal in treatment planning is to deliver the highest radiation dose to the malignant cells and the lowest dose to the nonmalignant tissues surrounding the tumor.[1]

The adverse effects of RT on normal tissues usually manifest as inflammatory changes.[1] RT total dose, fraction size, duration of radiation course, interval between fractions, dose rate, the involved organ, and the irradiated volume are the most important factors modulating the adverse effects of RT.[2] The response of the normal tissues to RT can be categorized into early or acute effects, occurring during the first days and weeks after RT, and late effects, which occur months, years, or even decades after treatment.[2] Some organs are more sensitive to the toxicity caused by acute effects and are called early responding tissues, whereas other tissues are prone to late toxic effects of RT and are called late responding tissues.[2]

Disclosure: The authors have nothing to disclose.
[a] Department of Radiology, Hospital of the University of Pennsylvania, 3400 Spruce Street, Philadelphia, PA 19104, USA; [b] Department of Gastroenterology, University of Pennsylvania, 3400 Spruce Street, Philadelphia, PA 19104, USA; [c] Department of Radiology, University of Minnesota, 420 Delaware Street SE, Minneapolis, MN 55455, USA; [d] Department of Radiation Oncology, University of Pennsylvania, 3400 Civic Boulevard, Philadelphia, PA 19104, USA
* Corresponding author. Hospital of the University of Pennsylvania, 3400 Spruce Street, Philadelphia, PA 19104.
E-mail address: abass.alavi@uphs.upenn.edu

Acute responses to radiation (early effects) are most prominently seen in tissues with large populations of cells with high turnover, such as bone marrow, skin, and mucosal surfaces of gastrointestinal and genitourinary tracts. Stem and progenitor cell pools in those tissues are depleted after irradiation, whereas differentiated and non-proliferating cells remain in the irradiated tissue and function until their normal turnover ends. Some tissues show subacute responses several months after RT, such as radiation pneumonitis (RP), radiation-induced liver injury, and Lhermitte syndrome. In this case, radiation affects cell populations with longer turnover time. Late effects of RT are generally less common but more severe with limited recovery. The affected cells in this type of injury are slowly proliferating cells, such as oligodendroglial or Schwann cells in the nervous tissue, tubular epithelium of kidneys, vascular endothelium, and fibroblasts. The late effects might take place decades after RT, such as atherosclerosis developing in survivors of breast cancer or lymphoma.[3] Breaks in the double strands of DNA causing micronuclei formation; chromosomal aberration; and loss of reproductive integrity of cell genome and eventually apoptosis and cell death are the main mechanisms of cell destruction by ionizing radiation.[4,5]

PET/computed tomography, especially fluorodeoxyglucose (FDG)-PET/CT, has been extensively used for diagnosis, prognostication, management, and assessment of response to treatment of various malignant lesions.[6–8] In addition, inflammatory cells have been shown to be FDG avid and detectable using FDG-PET/CT.[9–12] Inflammation induced by RT has been shown to be FDG avid and detectable by FDG-PET/CT.[1] This article discusses the role of the FDG-PET/CT imaging modality in assessment and prediction of complications of RT in various organ systems. **Table 1** summarizes the PET studies assessing the complications of RT.

RADIATION-INDUCED LUNG INFLAMMATION

One of the life-threatening early complications of RT is acute RP, an acute and subacute form of radiation-induced injury to the lung parenchyma happening after radiation in 4% to 30% of patients treated with curative intent.[2,13] The onset ranges from 1 to 6 months after RT, and the clinical syndrome includes nonproductive cough, dyspnea, fever, and pleuritic chest pain and rales.[14–16] Delayed radiation fibrosis occurs months to years after RT, and clinically significant fibrosis is more common in patients who developed acute RP.[17] With 30 to 70 Gy of RT, changes are evident in the radiographic images of 30% to 90% of cases. The volume of irradiated lung is another factor determining the occurrence of RP. Pulmonary function tests show decreased volumes and diffusion of the lung by the 16th week after RT.[18] Some of the biomarkers that are under investigation as predictors, although nonspecific, include serum surfactant apoprotein, interleukin (IL)-10, IL-6, and transforming growth factor beta.[19–25] Although the management of RP with high-dose steroid therapy usually results in rapid improvement of symptoms,[26] fatal RP has been reported to occur in up to 2% of patients receiving definitive chemoradiation for lung cancer.[13] Furthermore, the diagnosis of RP is challenging because of confounding medical factors, such as underlying malignancy, pulmonary edema, thromboembolic disease, and infection. The current clinical scoring systems used for diagnosis of RP do not yield accurate diagnosis in 28% to 48% of cases.[27,28]

Usefulness of FDG-PET/CT has been demonstrated in the assessment of lung inflammation in chronic obstructive pulmonary disease, sarcoidosis, bronchitis, and idiopathic interstitial pneumonia.[29–31] Some studies have investigated the role of FDG-PET/CT in assessment of radiation effects on the lung and its relationship with radiation dose.[32–36] Hicks and colleagues[34] qualitatively investigated the inflammatory changes in the lung parenchyma in 73 patients with non–small cell lung cancer (NSCLC) undergoing RT using FDG-PET/CT, compared them with the metabolic response of the tumor, and proposed a positive relationship between tumor radioresponsiveness and radiosensitivity of the normal tissue. Guerrero and colleagues[32] investigated 36 patients with esophageal cancer undergoing thoracic RT and restaging FDG-PET/CT after 4 to 12 weeks and found a linear relationship between regional radiation dose and voxel-averaged FDG uptake as a marker of RP response. They also found varying slopes for the radiation dose–FDG uptake plots, which were independent of the irradiated lung volume and the interval between RT and PET imaging. They suggested this slope, the pulmonary metabolic radiation dose response (PMRR), as a measure for assessment of intensity of RP. Echeverria and colleagues[37] used the same method for assessment of proton therapy–induced RP in patients with esophageal cancer and found a correlation between symptomatic patients and PMRR. Hart and colleagues,[33] in their retrospective study of 101 patients with esophageal cancer undergoing restaging FDG-PET/CT 3 to 12 weeks after RT, scored symptoms of RP in patients using National Institutes of Health Common Toxicity Criteria and showed an association between

Table 1
PET studies assessing the complications of RT

Disease	Complication	Author, Year	N	Clinical Setting	Finding and Conclusion
Lung cancer	RP	Abdulla et al,[36] 2014	20	Quantitative volumetric FDG-PET/CT parameters in patients with stage III NSCLC were calculated before and after RT (68.73 ± 6.92 Gy) and compared	In the lung with the primary tumor receiving RT, SUV_{mean} of the lung parenchyma and total lung parenchymal glycolysis increased after RT. The contralateral lung did not show significant changes. Global lung uptake parameters may be useful for quantification of lung inflammation
Lung cancer	Radiation esophagitis	Yuan et al,[91] 2014	50	Prospective study of patient with stage I–III NSCLC undergoing FDG-PET/CT before and during RT (≥60 Gy). Normalized SUV_{max} of esophagus to blood pool was measured and compared with symptomatic radiation esophagitis	16 patients developed symptoms in which the FDG uptake was significantly higher during RT compared with baseline (1.46 ± 0.12 vs 1.11 ± 0.05; $P = .002$)
Lung cancer	Cardiac toxicity	Evans at al,[65] 2013	39	Patients with lung malignancies close to the heart and treated with SBRT (<50 Gy in 4 fractions) underwent FDG-PET/CT imaging before and after therapy and were assessed qualitatively	9 of the 19 patients receiving 20 Gy to >5 cm of the heart had increased FDG uptake vs 0 out of 20 patients having <5 cm irradiated with 20 Gy ($P = .0004$)
Lung cancer, esophageal cancer, multiple myeloma, gastric cancer	Cardiac toxicity	Unal et al,[62] 2013	38	Patients with thoracic malignancy treated with RT (median dose of 64 Gy (30–76 Gy), daily fractional dose 2.0 Gy) and FDG-PET/CT scans at least 3 mo after RT were assessed for myocardial FDG uptake qualitatively and quantitatively (SUV_{max})	Significantly higher glucose metabolism in the irradiated myocardium vs intact myocardium. SUV_{max}, SUV_{min}, SUV_{mean} were 21.5, 3.3, and 8.8 for irradiated and 6, 1.3, and 3 for nonirradiated myocardium ($P<.001$)
Lung cancer	RP	McCurdy et al,[120] 2012	24	Assessment of the dose response in patients with lung cancer using post-RT FDG-PET/CT. Patients received restaging PET/CT 4–12 wk after RT. Histogram analysis was performed and the slope of voxel average FDG-PET vs radiation dose was calculated (PMRR). Common Toxicity Criteria version 3 was used for scoring clinical symptoms. Various parameters were assessed using ROC curve analysis to predict clinical outcomes	A linear relationship between radiation dose and FDG uptake was found, for which its slope might be used as a surrogate marker for RP

(continued on next page)

Table 1
(continued)

Disease	Complication	Author, Year	N	Clinical Setting	Finding and Conclusion
Lung cancer	RP	Petit et al,[121] 2011	101	To test the hypothesis that pretreatment inflammation in the lung makes the lung more susceptible to RP. The relationship between FDG uptake of the lung, radiation dose, and RILT was assessed. Once or twice daily 1.5, 1.8, or 2 Gy. Total dose 28.5–79.2 Gy	Univariate logistic regression showed that increased lung density and pretreatment FDG uptake were related to post-RT RILT. The 95th percentile of the FDG uptake (P = .016; OR = 4.3), age (P = .029, OR = 1.06), and pre-RT dyspnea score of ≥1 (P = .005; OR = 0.20) were significant in the multivariable logistic regression. The risk of RILT increased with 95th percentile of pre-RT FDG uptake. Decreasing the irradiation exposure to normal areas can reduce the risk of RILT
Lung cancer	RP	Mac Manus et al,[14] 2011	88	FDG-PET was performed after RT (median 70 d) and platinum-based chemoradiation therapy in 15 cases (60 Gy in 30 fractions). RT-induced inflammation was qualitatively graded by blinded observer. RP was graded using RTOG scale blindly	Significant association between worst RP grade at any time and FDG radiotoxicity grade (1-sided P = .033). The worst RTOG score after PET was also associated with PET radiotoxicity grade (1-sided P = .035). Visual scoring of the FDG uptake was correlated with presence and severity of RP
Lung cancer	RP	De Ruysscher et al,[122] 2009	18	FDG-PET/CT scans were obtained 0, 7, and 14 d after RT in patients with stage III NSCLC. SUV_{max} was assessed and serum IL-6 was also measured at the mentioned time points. RILT was measured based on clinical scores	There was no significant difference in FDG uptake among patients with or without RILT before RT; however, the group that developed RILT had significantly increased FDG uptake on days 7 and 14 post-RT. IL-6 and mean lung dose were not correlated with RILT
Lung cancer	RP	Hicks et al,[34] 2004	73	Qualitative assessment of the inflammatory changes in the lung parenchyma in patients with NSCLC undergoing radical RT using FDG-PET/CT and comparing with metabolic response of the tumor	Positive relationship between tumor radioresponsiveness and radiosensitivity of the normal tissue based on the genetic determinants for sensitivity of the normal tissue

		Author et al, Year	N	Methods	Results
Esophageal cancer	RP	McCurdy et al,[123] 2013	75	Patients treated with chemoradiation who underwent restaging FDG-PET/CT 1–3 mo after treatment were included. Common Terminology Criteria for Adverse Events were used for scoring of pneumonitis. Radiation dose and FDG uptake were calculated in the upper lobe and lower lobe. PMRR was calculated for each region	Upper lung lobes had higher PMRR vs lower lobes. A higher ratio of mean dose to the lower lung lobes and higher SUV in the region receiving 0–10 Gy to the entire lung predicted pneumonitis
Esophageal cancer	RP	Echeverria et al,[37] 2013	100	Patients with esophageal cancer treated with proton therapy. PMRR was quantified as the slope of normalized FDG uptake in lung tissue vs radiation dose	Significant correlation between PMRR and RP clinical scores was observed. PMRR was 0.022 for the symptomatic group and 0.012 in the nonsymptomatic group ($P = .014$)
Esophageal cancer	Cardiac toxicity	Konski et al,[124] 2012	102	Patients with esophageal cancer undergoing chemoradiation (median dose, 50.5 Gy [45–57.6 Gy] in 1.8-Gy fractions) were assessed for symptomatic cardiac toxicity. Radiation dosimetry, demographic factors and FDG-PET uptake in the myocardium were calculated and correlated with cardiac toxicity measured by RTOG and CTCAE v3.0	In 12 patients with treatment-related cardiac toxicity, 6 were symptomatic. In comparison, of symptomatic and asymptomatic groups, mean heart V20, V30, and V40 were significantly higher in the group with symptoms ($P<.05$). No correlation was found between FDG uptake and cardiac toxicity. Women were the most affected subgroup of patients
Esophageal cancer	RP	Hart et al,[33] 2008	101	The relationship between RP clinical symptoms and FDG uptake was assessed. Patients with esophageal cancer underwent FDG-PET 3–12 wk after RT. Normalized FDG vs radiation dose plot was drawn and PMRR was calculated. Mean lung dose, percentage of the lung receiving >20 Gy, and RP outcomes were correlated with clinical outcomes	Increased values of both MLD and PMRR were associated with higher probability of RP clinical symptoms ($P = .032$, $P = .033$, respectively). The combination of MLD and PMRR was superior to MLD or PMRR alone for assessment of RP
Esophageal cancer	RP	Guerrero et al,[32] 2007	36	Assessment of the relationship between local radiation dose received by the lung and FDG-PET uptake. Patients with esophageal cancer underwent PET/CT 4–12 wk after RT. Voxel-based analysis was used for correlation	Regional radiation dose and voxel-averaged FDG uptake had a linear relationship. The slopes of the radiation dose–FDG uptake plot varied among patients

(continued on next page)

Table 1
(continued)

Disease	Complication	Author, Year	N	Clinical Setting	Finding and Conclusion
Esophageal cancer	Cardiac toxicity	Jingu et al,[64] 2006	64	Assessment of focal increased FDG uptake in basal myocardium of patients with esophageal cancer undergoing RT (2 Gy fractional daily dose 5 d a wk up to 30–70 Gy) and FDG-PET/CT >3 mo after RT and correlation with SPECT and MR imaging	Increased FDG uptake was often seen in the irradiated myocardium, which might indicate RT-induced damage to the heart
Head and neck cancer	Vascular inflammation	Wang et al,[68] 2013	17	Patients with stage III to IVA pharyngeal cancer underwent chemoradiation therapy (36–45 Gy), FDG-PET/CT before treatment and 1 mo after the start of therapy, and carotid arteries were assessed for increased FDG uptake (SUV_{max} and TBR)	Significant increase in the TBR 1 mo after treatment in both carotids ($P<.002$) and also the aorta. SUV_{max} showed a similar pattern of increase after treatment. The results suggest that cisplatin-based chemoradiation triggers systemic vascular inflammation that might progress to atherosclerosis
Head and neck cancer	Parotid gland injury	Cannon et al,[111] 2012	98	Quantitative measurement of parotid FDG uptake for assessment of xerostomia after RT (66–70 Gy in fractions of 30–35) was done in this study using baseline and post-RT FDG-PET/CT and voxel-based analysis. D_{Met} was defined as pretreatment parotid SUV/dose and used for prediction of parotid injury after RT	Loss of parotid FDG uptake correlated with clinical symptoms of parotid toxicity. D_{Met} was able to accurately predict post-RT changes in the parotid gland

Head and neck cancer	Soft tissue injury	Dornfeld et al,[125] 2008	27	Assessment of inflammation in the normal soft tissues caused by RT (2-Gy daily fractions to 66–74 Gy) in patients with head and neck cancer using FDG-PET/CT at 3 and 12 mo after RT	SUV levels in the normal soft tissues and glottic area at 12 mo after RT were associated with lower quality of life and restricted diet. SUV levels 3 mo after RT did not show this correlation. This study showed that abnormal metabolism in the irradiated tissues persists up to 1 y after RT
Cranial ALL	Neurocognitive function decline	Krull et al,[82] 2014	38	Association between regional brain metabolism and neurocognitive outcome in the adult survivors of childhood ALL having cranial radiation (19 patients 18 Gy, 19 patients 24 Gy) was assessed using FDG-PET/CT and neurocognitive tests	The survivors showed lower cognitive function compared with normal subjects (P<.001). Basal ganglia structures had higher activity in the group irradiated with 24 Gy. This study suggested decreased efficacy of frontostriatal brain circuit in ALL survivors
CNS tumor	Neurocognitive decline	Hahn et al,[81] 2009	11	Prospective study to relate the radiologically defined dose-dependent changes in the brain to cognitive function of patients with primary tumors of brain or cerebral meninges. FDG and 15O-PET and neuropsychological tests were done before, 3 wk after, and 6 mo after RT (1.8–2 Gy/daily fractions; 50–60 Gy in 5–6 wk). Regional radiation dose, follow-up time and neuropsychological tests were correlated with PET uptake	6 out of 11 patients completed the study. FDG-PET showed 2%–6% decreases in the areas receiving >40 Gy at third week and sixth month. 15O-PET showed <10% increase in the relative regional blood flow in areas of brain receiving >30 Gy and decrease at 6-mo follow-up. There was a dose-dependent metabolic response in CNS tissue. Decreased FDG uptake was correlated with decreased neuropsychological performance in problem solving, cognitive flexibility, and global measures of psychological disorder

Abbreviations: ALL, acute lymphoblastic leukemia; CNS, central nervous system; CTCAE v3.0, Common Terminology Criteria for Adverse Events, Version 3.0; IL, interleukin; MLD, mean lung dose; NSCLC, non–small cell lung cancer; OR, odds ratio; PMRR, pulmonary metabolic radiation dose response; RILT, radiation-induced lung toxicity; RP, radiation pneumonitis; ROC, receiver operating characteristic; RTOG, Radiation Therapy Oncology Group; SBRT, stereotactic body radiation therapy; SPECT, single-photon emission computed tomography; TBR, tissue to background ratio; V20, lung volume receiving ≥20 Gy; V30, lung volume receiving ≥30 Gy; V40, lung volume receiving ≥40 Gy.

increase in the mean lung radiation dose and FDG uptake and RP (*P* = .032 for mean lung radiation dose, *P* = .033 for FDG uptake, respectively).

Recently, in a pilot study of 20 patients, Abdulla and colleagues[36] quantified the global lung parenchymal FDG uptake after RT in patients with stage III NSCLC by subtracting the tumor uptake from the total lung FDG uptake using volume-based quantitative FDG-PET/CT parameters. They found statistically significant increases in global lung uptake parameters such as global lung glycolysis, total lesion glycolysis (TLG), and lung parenchyma mean standardized uptake value (SUV$_{mean}$) in the irradiated lung and no significant changes in the nonirradiated lung. This study showed the ability of volumetric PET parameters to be potential biomarkers for assessment of lung inflammation after RT (**Figs. 1** and **2**).

The emergence of proton therapy, which provides improvements in localization of radiation dose and reductions in delivered dose to normal tissues, may allow for fewer treatment toxicities, specifically radiation-induced lung injury, and an increase in effectiveness of treatment compared with photon therapy.[38–42] Further studies are needed to more precisely evaluate the post-RT changes in the lungs using FDG-PET/CT.

CARDIAC COMPLICATIONS

Another common cause for morbidity and mortality after RT is cardiovascular sequelae.[43] Heart complications are most commonly reported as developing 10 to 15 years after RT and the usual cardiac risk factors, such as obesity, hypertension, and smoking, aggravate the disease.[2] There is a wide range of cardiovascular complications following RT, including coronary artery disease (CAD), valvular disease, pericarditis, cardiomyopathy, autonomic dysfunction, vascular changes, and arrhythmia.[43,44]

Effect of Radiation Therapy on Ischemic Heart Disease Mortality in Patients with Cancer

There is an increase in the incidence of CAD among patients with cancer treated with thoracic RT, who have fairly long survival times, such as for breast cancer and Hodgkin lymphoma.[45–48] RT for breast cancer might increase the incidence

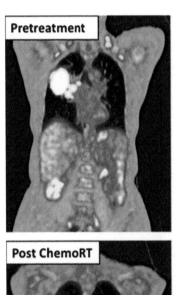
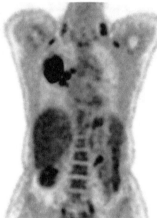
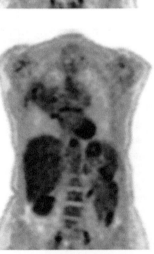

Fig. 1. Radiation-induced lung inflammation. The top row shows a primary non–small cell lung cancer with lymph node involvement (*left,* CT scan fused with FDG-PET; *right,* PET-only image) before treatment. The bottom row shows the same patient after chemoradiation with resultant inflammatory changes in the lung parenchyma (*left,* CT scan fused with FDG-PET; *right,* PET-only image). ChemoRT, chemoradiation therapy.

Pretreatment

Post ChemoRT

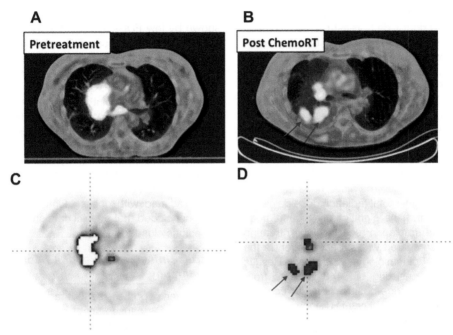

Fig. 2. Assessment of response to treatment in a patient with non–small cell lung cancer. Pretreatment PET study (*A, C*) shows the primary tumor. Posttreatment study (*B, D*) shows a decrease in the size of the tumor and appearance of a new avidity in the posterior portion of the lung parenchyma adjunct to the primary lesion (*red arrows*), most likely caused by inflammation in the lung from RT. Quantitative assessment of the lung lesions and the corresponding PET parameters, such as metabolic tumor volume (MTV), SUV_{max}, SUV_{mean}, partial volume corrected SUV_{mean} ($pvcSUV_{mean}$), TLG, partial volume corrected TLG (pvcTLG), and SUV_{peak}, are shown in the table (*E*).

	MTV	SUVmax	SUVmean	pvcSUVmean	TLG	pvcTLG	SUVpeak
Primary tumor before treatment	49.8	12.7	7.5	10.6	372.4	631.6	11.2
Lymph node before treatment	3.9	7.1	4.3	7.7	16.7	28.6	5.8
Primary tumor after treatment	1.8	6.4	4.5	7.9	8	13.2	5.3
Lymph node after treatment	1.2	4.9	3.9	7.1	4.5	7.4	4.2
New lesion, most likely inflammation	35.6	4.5	3	3.9	107.1	159.2	4.1

of ischemic heart disease, mostly because of the anatomic proximity of the radiation site to the heart, and particularly to the left anterior descending artery.[49–51] Various studies have investigated the linkage between RT and long-term cardiovascular mortality.[3,50–57] Rutqvist and colleagues,[55] in their 16-year follow-up of 960 women with early stage breast cancer less than 71 years old who received surgery and RT to 45 Gy in 5 weeks versus surgery alone, found a 3-fold higher mortality risk caused by ischemic heart disease in patients with higher radiation doses. Ragaz and colleagues,[53] in a 20-year follow-up of 318 women, found a slight increase in the risk of cardiovascular mortality in 2 groups of patients: those undergoing mastectomy alone, and those undergoing mastectomy plus RT.

One of the most prominent studies is by Darby and colleagues,[3] which assessed major coronary events such as coronary revascularization, myocardial infarction, and death caused by ischemic heart disease in 2168 female patients (963 patients with major coronary event and 1205 controls) undergoing RT for breast cancer between 1958 and 2001. The rate of major coronary events was linearly correlated with the mean dose to the heart (7.4% increase per gray) irrespective of preexisting cardiac risk factors. Higher rates of major coronary events were observed in women with left-sided breast cancer. Having a history of ischemic heart disease imposed a higher risk (odds ratio [OR] = 6.67) for major coronary events. The investigators concluded that clinicians might need to consider cardiac risk factors in their treatment decision and plan. In contrast, Hojris and colleagues,[54] in a 12-year follow-up of 3083 patients less than 70 years old with breast cancer, did not find any difference in rates of ischemic heart disease between 2 randomly assigned groups receiving or not receiving RT after mastectomy. In addition, Rutter and colleagues,[56] in a more recent large cohort of 344,831 patients from 1998 to 2006, noted no difference between left-sided and right-sided breast cancer in overall survival. Therefore, they concluded that the importance of cardiac-related complications is less than previously shown, likely because of the improvements in RT techniques in the last decades.

Although the risk of radiation-induced cardiac toxicity among patients with breast cancer is a late effect that may be minimal to negligible with the use of modern treatment planning techniques, cardiac toxicity for patients receiving RT for lung cancer remains a clinical concern in both the subacute and late settings. The difference may be explained by the higher total radiation dose delivered for treatment and the significantly higher mean heart doses of irradiation received when treating lung cancer compared with breast cancer. In the Surveillance, Epidemiology, and End Results (SEER) study consisting of 6148 patients from 1983 to 1993 with node-positive NSCLC receiving surgical resection plus adjuvant RT, increased cardiac disease mortality was noted in patients treated with postoperative RT (hazard ratio, 1.30; 95% confidence interval, 1.04–1.61; $P = .0193$).[58] Even with modern treatment techniques, radiation-induced cardiac mortality may remain prevalent. In a 2015 report from the Radiation Therapy Oncology Group, among 544 patients with locally advanced NSCLC treated with definitive chemoradiation to 2 dose levels, at a median follow-up of only 22 months, dose to the heart on multivariate analysis significant influenced overall survival ($P = .0035$).[59]

Further studies and meta-analyses and systematic reviews are needed to elucidate the exact effect of RT on CAD mortality. FDG-PET/CT has been shown to be an independent biomarker for prediction of heart disease and atherosclerosis.[60] Almost all of the patients undergoing RT currently have at least 1 PET/CT scan in their records, so it might be useful to assess the effect of RT in the development of CAD in this group of patients and aid the findings of the abovementioned studies.

Myocardial Changes and PET/Computed Tomography

Severe cardiomyopathies can also occur as late effects of RT. RT's main target in injury of the heart, unlike chemotherapeutic agents, is thought to be the endothelial cell population, which adversely affects the vasculoconnective stroma of the myocardium.[61] Diffuse interstitial fibrosis is the consequence of RT in the myocardium. However, it is rare to cause damage to myocardium with therapeutic doses of radiation.[2]

The effect of RT on the myocardium has been shown by few FDG-PET/CT studies[62–64] and has been described as focal FDG uptake in the basal myocardium[64] or unusual sharp borders excluding the apex.[63] Unal and colleagues,[62] who visually investigated FDG-PET/CT images of 28 patients for regional myocardial uptake 4 months after RT, observed annular or focal increased FDG uptake in the irradiated myocardium. Evans and colleagues[65] reviewed FDG-PET/CT of 39 patients treated with stereotactic body RT of the tumors close to the heart and found increased FDG uptake in the heart when more than 5 cm^3 of the heart was irradiated with doses of more than 20 Gy. They concluded that special care should be taken for lesions close to the heart.

Vascular Inflammation and PET/Computed Tomography

It has been hypothesized that radiation to the coronary arteries causes latent injuries to the capillaries of the endothelial cells and leads to cytoplasmic swelling and thrombosis. As a result, there is rapid proliferation of the endothelium, which leads to ischemia and myocardial fibrosis.[61] Increase in the dose of each fraction is related to increased risk of CAD. With increases in the volume of the irradiated heart, the minimum dose for causing damage decreases.

FDG-PET/CT has been shown to be a promising surrogate marker for vascular inflammation and atherosclerosis.[66,67] Wang and colleagues[68] assessed the applicability of PET/CT in assessment of vascular inflammation induced by RT and cisplatin chemotherapy in the systemic and local vascular system. They performed serial PET/CT scans on 17 patients before and during chemoradiation therapy for head and neck cancers and assessed the carotid arteries for FDG-avid lesions. They observed a general trend of increasing FDG uptake (tissue to background ratio (TBR) and SUV$_{max}$) not only in local arteries such as carotids, ascending aorta, aortic arch, and descending aorta but also at more remote sites such as abdominal aorta and even iliac arteries ($P<.006$ for TBR). They concluded that the inflammation seen in the vessels after chemoradiation might be responsible for the increased rate of atheroembolic accident after chemoradiation and that PET/CT might be able to predict such risk.

EFFECT OF RADIATION ON THE CENTRAL NERVOUS SYSTEM

The effect of RT on the central nervous system (CNS) has been described as acute, early delayed, or late delayed.[35] In acute radiation encephalopathy the changes occur days to weeks after RT. Early-delayed changes occur 1 to 6 months after RT and consist of transient demyelination and somnolence that may most prominently affect children. These reactions resolve in 1 to 3 months and are not predictive of late complications.[69] Late-delayed effects consist of demyelination, vascular changes, and white matter necrosis[70] occurring more than 6 months after RT with high doses.[69,71] The response of the CNS to RT is initially increased intracranial pressure caused by the edema in neural tissues. Headache, nausea, somnolence, neurocognitive deficits, motor-sensory deficits, and seizures can develop from this increased intracranial pressure. After subacute phases, presentations such as brain necrosis caused by infarction and gliosis appear.[2] RT-induced intellectual deterioration, even with a low total dose, affects hippocampal-dependent functions such as learning, memory, and spatial information.[72] Up to 50% of long-term survivor adult patients with partial or whole-brain irradiation present with cognitive impairment, such as acute memory loss or dementia.[73–75]

Fractional whole-brain irradiation in animal models and calculation of local rates of glucose metabolism in different functional tasks has been reported.[76] The PET studies comparing preirradiation and postirradiation brain function using specific functional tasks have revealed the imbalance in different regions of the brain, including frontal subcortical areas, dorsal prefrontal cortex, hippocampus, cuneate, and motor areas.[77,78]

In early studies, it was reported that the RT does not alter the metabolic activity of the brain.[79,80] Kahkonen and colleagues[80] assessed the posttherapy FDG-PET of 44 acute lymphoblastic leukemia (ALL) long-term survivors and found no difference between 2 groups. Hahn and colleagues[81] prospectively studied the relationship between dose-dependent radiologic changes in the brains of patients with primary tumors of the brain or cerebral meninges undergoing RT with neurocognitive decline using FDG and O-H_2O PET and found a 2% to 6% FDG decrease in the regions of brain receiving more than 40 Gy in 2 follow-up intervals of 3 weeks and 6 months, whereas O-H_2O showed increases in 2 follow-up intervals when greater than 30 Gy was delivered. There was also a significant correlation between FDG decrease and neuropsychological decline. Krull and colleagues[82] compared the FDG-PET–measured regional brain metabolism with the neurocognitive outcomes of long-term ALL survivors undergoing RT of the head and noted an association with increased metabolic activity in the frontal lobe cortex and basal ganglia, which suggests compromise of the frontostriatal brain circuit.

RADIATION-INDUCED ESOPHAGITIS

RT-induced odynophagia and dysphagia are acute symptoms most likely caused by abnormal peristalsis, mucositis, focal erosions, and ulcerations.[83] Abnormal peristalsis and dysphagia may continue for months after RT. Strictures caused by submucosal fibrosis occur in 1% to 5% of patients treated with definitive thoracic RT and develop 3 to 18 months after RT. It has been shown that the incidence of esophageal late effects was 6% in patients treated with 60 Gy for 6 weeks after surgery, whereas another group of patients had 1% incidence when treated with 50 Gy for 5 weeks before surgery.[84]

Several studies have reported a relationship between radiation esophagitis and the increase in the FDG uptake in patients treated for esophageal[85–88] and lung cancers.[89,90] The latest study is by Yuan and colleagues,[91] which prospectively investigated whether the changes in the esophageal FDG uptake before and during RT are related to the symptoms of the radiation esophagitis in 50 patients with stage I to III NSCLC and noted an increase in the normalized SUV uptake during RT at the tumor level (1.09 ± 0.05 vs 1.28 ± 0.06; $P = .001$), which might serve as a predicting factor for esophagitis. Nijkamp and colleagues[90] correlated the RT dose with the acute esophagitis clinical scores by using FDG parameters in patients with NSCLC undergoing concurrent chemoradiation. They showed an association between FDG uptake and acute esophagitis grade. Twenty-five patients with grade less than 2 and 57 patients with grade greater than or equal to 2 were compared and the top 50% of SUV values ($SUV_{50\%}$) were higher in the group with grade greater than or equal to 2 (2.2 vs 2.6; $P<.01$). In addition, local dose effect relation was established between planned dose and FDG uptake of posttreatment PET scans (>55 Gy indicated increase in the uptake of FDG). These studies show the ability of esophageal FDG uptake in prediction of the severity of acute esophagitis after RT or concurrent chemotherapy.

PET/COMPUTED TOMOGRAPHY FOR EVALUATION OF INSUFFICIENCY FRACTURES

One of the subtypes of stress fracture is insufficiency fracture (IF), which happens when the normal or physiologic stress causes fracture in a demineralized bone or bone with decreased elastic resistance.[92] Several factors contribute to IF, including osteoporosis, steroid and bisphosphonate use, rheumatoid arthritis, and RT.[93–95] IF has been reported after RT to the pelvis in gynecologic,[96–103] prostate, anal, and rectal cancers.[100] IF can cause severe pain mimicking the pain of bone metastasis.

FDG-PET/CT has been used for assessment of IF after RT.[92] However, there are only a limited number of cases reporting findings of IF using this modality.[104–108] The findings of IF in PET images include variable degrees of uptake depending on several factors, including the interval between fracture and PET imaging, age of the patient, and the affected bone.[109] Therefore, special attention should be paid in the clinic to prevent misdiagnosis of this finding.[108] In addition, Kato and colleagues[109] evaluated FDG-PET/CT for differentiation of benign and malignant fractures in 20 selected patients having FDG-PET/CT scans and with evidence of fractures and found a statistically significant differences between benign (SUV of 1.36 ± 0.49) and malignant (SUV of $4.46 \pm .2.12$, $P<.01$) groups and suggested FDG-PET/CT as a useful differentiator of benign and malignant metastatic fractures.

SALIVARY GLAND INJURY AFTER RADIATION THERAPY

Salivary gland injury can occur with RT for head and neck tumors. Xerostomia caused by salivary gland insufficiency can cause chewing, speech, and swallowing problems and dental cavities.[110] RT dose, the percentage of irradiated gland, and function of the parotid before RT determine the incidence of clinical symptoms.[111–113] Acute xerostomia caused by RT improves within months after RT and the parotid gland's activity improves over years.[114] Significant parotid sparing happens with doses of less than 24 Gy or 26 Gy for stimulated or unstimulated flow, respectively.[115] Because the parotid gland secretes 60% of the saliva, most of the studies focus on the parotid gland.

PET studies based on ^{11}C-methionine and FDG have been used to investigate the effects of RT on the parotid glands.[79,111,116] Imaging with ^{11}C-methionin PET shows decreased ^{11}C-methionine uptake in irradiated parotid glands.[117] Roach and colleagues[116] retrospectively assessed preradiation and postradiation FDG-PET of 49 patients with head and neck squamous cell carcinoma undergoing intensity-modulated RT and found a dose relationship with a linear pattern for SUV_{mean} and sigmoidal decline for SUV_{max} with increasing dose of radiation. Xerostomia, being one of the major complications of parotid injury during head and neck RT, has been investigated by Cannon and colleagues[111] to evaluate the potential of quantitative FDG-PET parameters as useful biomarkers for xerostomia after RT. Ninety-eight patients with head and neck cancers who received definitive RT were included and RT dose and SUV uptake of the parotids were calculated before and after RT. Pretreatment parotid gland SUV weighted by dose was able to predict the posttreatment changes in the parotid FDG uptake (ie, fractional parotid SUV). The loss of FDG uptake was correlated with posttreatment early parotid toxicity ($P<.01$). The investigators concluded that dose-weighted pretreatment parotid SUV might potentially be used for treatment planning.

PET/COMPUTED TOMOGRAPHY AS A PREDICTOR OF HEMATOLOGICAL TOXICITY AFTER RADIATION THERAPY

Bone marrow (BM) often receives incidental irradiation during RT for a variety of malignancies.[2] The extent of the complications depends on the amount of BM reserve, the exposed volume of BM, and history of chemotherapy. Restoration of BM after RT depends mostly on volume of BM irradiated and RT dose received.

Rose and colleagues[118] investigated PET/CT as a metabolic biomarker for hematological toxicity in patients undergoing RT. Elicin and colleagues[119] quantified FDG uptake and volume of BM of patients with cervical cancer treated with chemoradiation therapy using PET/CT. They related differences of pretherapy and posttherapy FDG uptake to hematological toxicity and found correlations between reduction of white blood cells and FDG uptake, even after low doses of radiation during chemoradiation therapy, 3 months after (r^2, 0.27; $P = .04$) and at the last follow-up (r^2, 0.25; $P = .04$). This study shows the usefulness of FDG-PET in predicting hematological toxicity and its possible use as a predictor of hematological complications of RT.

SUMMARY

This article discusses the role of PET/CT imaging in the assessment of early and late complications of RT. In addition to the diagnostic, prognostic, staging, and treatment follow-up and planning roles of PET/CT in different cancers, detection and prediction of adverse effects of RT are potentially important aspects of PET/CT imaging. For example, detection of RP, sometimes challenged by using other clinical criteria, might be aided by accurate and quantitative PET parameters before or after RT. FDG-PET/CT has also been shown to be feasible for the assessment of cardiovascular adverse events such as vascular inflammation and cardiomyopathies. Future studies focusing on specific cancers and irradiated organs are needed to clarify the role of PET/CT imaging in assessment of RT and chemotherapy complications.

However, currently the literature regarding some of these complications is scarce and most of the studies have been limited to reporting just correlations between PET parameters and occurrence of complications. Therefore, there is a knowledge gap regarding applicability of PET/CT as a predictive tool for RT and chemotherapy complications. Further studies would resolve this limitation and clarify the role of PET/CT in the assessment of RT and chemotherapy complications.

One of the challenges in the application of PET/CT as a tool for assessment and prognostication of RT and chemotherapy complications is the cost of this imaging modality. PET/CT has a major impact on patients with malignant diseases and has increased the efficiency of diagnosis and treatment of these patients. As a result, patients with various types of cancer, such as lung, pancreatic, esophageal, lymphoma, and melanoma, have at least 1 or 2 PET/CT studies as routine procedures in their diagnosis, treatment, and follow-up that could be used for investigation of the complications of RT.

In conclusion, we think that the information available in the currently acquired PET images of patients with cancer in the baseline and follow-up sessions is valuable regarding the effects of RT on the human body and the evolution of the short-term and long-term complications of RT and chemotherapy.

REFERENCES

1. Ulaner GA, Lyall A. Identifying and distinguishing treatment effects and complications from malignancy at FDG PET/CT. Radiographics 2013;33(6): 1817–34.
2. Perez CA. Principles and practice of radiation oncology. 5th edition. Philadelphia: Lippincott Williams & Wilkins; 2008.
3. Darby SC, Ewertz M, McGale P, et al. Risk of ischemic heart disease in women after radiotherapy for breast cancer. N Engl J Med 2013; 368(11):987–98.
4. Alper T. Cellular radiobiology. London: University Press; 1979.
5. Elkind MM, Whitmore GF. The radiobiology of cultured mammalian cells. New York: Gordon & Breach; 1967.
6. Hess S, Blomberg BA, Zhu HJ, et al. The pivotal role of FDG-PET/CT in modern medicine. Acad Radiol 2014;21(2):232–49.

7. Xanthopoulos EP, Corradetti MN, Mitra N, et al. Impact of PET staging in limited-stage small-cell lung cancer. J Thorac Oncol 2013;8(7):899–905.
8. Geiger GA, Kim MB, Xanthopoulos EP, et al. Stage migration in planning PET/CT scans in patients due to receive radiotherapy for non-small-cell lung cancer. Clin Lung Cancer 2014;15(1):79–85.
9. Basu S, Zhuang H, Torigian DA, et al. Functional imaging of inflammatory diseases using nuclear medicine techniques. Semin Nucl Med 2009; 39(2):124–45.
10. Houshmand S, Salavati A, Hess S, et al. An update on novel quantitative techniques in the context of evolving whole-body PET imaging. PET Clin 2015; 10(1):45–58.
11. Houshmand S, Salavati A, Basu S, et al. The role of dual and multiple time point imaging of FDG uptake in both normal and disease states. Clin Translational Imaging 2014;2(4):281–93.
12. Cheng G, Torigian DA, Zhuang H, et al. When should we recommend use of dual time-point and delayed time-point imaging techniques in FDG PET? Eur J Nucl Med Mol Imaging 2013;40(5): 779–87.
13. Palma DA, Senan S, Tsujino K, et al. Predicting radiation pneumonitis after chemoradiation therapy for lung cancer: an international individual patient data meta-analysis. Int J Radiat Oncol Biol Phys 2013;85(2):444–50.
14. Mac Manus MP, Ding Z, Hogg A, et al. Association between pulmonary uptake of fluorodeoxyglucose detected by positron emission tomography scanning after radiation therapy for non-small-cell lung cancer and radiation pneumonitis. Int J Radiat Oncol Biol Phys 2011;80(5):1365–71.
15. Abratt RP, Morgan GW, Silvestri G, et al. Pulmonary complications of radiation therapy. Clin Chest Med 2004;25(1):167–77.
16. Gross NJ. Pulmonary effects of radiation therapy. Ann Intern Med 1977;86(1):81–92.
17. Mazeron R, Etienne-Mastroianni B, Pérol D, et al. Predictive factors of late radiation fibrosis: a prospective study in non-small cell lung cancer. Int J Radiat Oncol Biol Phys 2010;77(1):38–43.
18. Marks LB, Spencer DP, Bentel GC, et al. The utility of SPECT lung perfusion scans in minimizing and assessing the physiologic consequences of thoracic irradiation. Int J Radiat Oncol Biol Phys 1993;26(4):659–68.
19. Anscher MS, Kong FM, Andrews K, et al. Plasma transforming growth factor beta1 as a predictor of radiation pneumonitis. Int J Radiat Oncol Biol Phys 1998;41(5):1029–35.
20. Anscher MS, Marks LB, Shafman TD, et al. Using plasma transforming growth factor beta-1 during radiotherapy to select patients for dose escalation. J Clin Oncol 2001;19(17):3758–65.

21. Arpin D, Perol D, Blay JY, et al. Early variations of circulating interleukin-6 and interleukin-10 levels during thoracic radiotherapy are predictive for radiation pneumonitis. J Clin Oncol 2005;23(34): 8748–56.

22. Barthelemy-Brichant N, Bosquée L, Cataldo D, et al. Increased IL-6 and TGF-beta1 concentrations in bronchoalveolar lavage fluid associated with thoracic radiotherapy. Int J Radiat Oncol Biol Phys 2004;58(3):758–67.

23. Chen Y, Rubin P, Williams J, et al. Circulating IL-6 as a predictor of radiation pneumonitis. Int J Radiat Oncol Biol Phys 2001;49(3):641–8.

24. Marks LB, Munley MT, Bentel GC, et al. Physical and biological predictors of changes in whole-lung function following thoracic irradiation. Int J Radiat Oncol Biol Phys 1997;39(3):563–70.

25. McDonald S, Meyerowitz C, Smudzin T, et al. Preliminary results of a pilot study using WR-2721 before fractionated irradiation of the head and neck to reduce salivary gland dysfunction. Int J Radiat Oncol Biol Phys 1994;29(4):747–54.

26. Delanian S, Balla-Mekias S, Lefaix JL. Striking regression of chronic radiotherapy damage in a clinical trial of combined pentoxifylline and tocopherol. J Clin Oncol 1999;17(10):3283–90.

27. Kocak Z, Evans ES, Zhou SM, et al. Challenges in defining radiation pneumonitis in patients with lung cancer. Int J Radiat Oncol Biol Phys 2005;62(3): 635–8.

28. Yirmibesoglu E, Higginson DS, Fayda M, et al. Challenges scoring radiation pneumonitis in patients irradiated for lung cancer. Lung Cancer 2012;76(3):350–3.

29. Kwee TC, Torigian DA, Alavi A. Nononcological applications of positron emission tomography for evaluation of the thorax. J Thorac Imaging 2013; 28(1):25–39.

30. Subramanian DR, Jenkins L, Edgar R, et al. Assessment of pulmonary neutrophilic inflammation in emphysema by quantitative positron emission tomography. Am J Respir Crit Care Med 2012;186(11):1125–32.

31. Torigian DA, Dam V, Chen X, et al. In vivo quantification of pulmonary inflammation in relation to emphysema severity via partial volume corrected (18)F-FDG-PET using computer-assisted analysis of diagnostic chest CT. Hell J Nucl Med 2013; 16(1):12–8.

32. Guerrero T, Johnson V, Hart J, et al. Radiation pneumonitis: local dose versus [18F]-fluorodeoxyglucose uptake response in irradiated lung. Int J Radiat Oncol Biol Phys 2007;68(4):1030–5.

33. Hart JP, McCurdy MR, Ezhil M, et al. Radiation pneumonitis: correlation of toxicity with pulmonary metabolic radiation response. Int J Radiat Oncol Biol Phys 2008;71(4):967–71.

34. Hicks RJ, Mac Manus MP, Matthews JP, et al. Early FDG-PET imaging after radical radiotherapy for non-small-cell lung cancer: inflammatory changes in normal tissues correlate with tumor response and do not confound therapeutic response evaluation. Int J Radiat Oncol Biol Phys 2004;60(2):412–8.

35. Robbins ME, Brunso-Bechtold JK, Peiffer AM, et al. Imaging radiation-induced normal tissue injury. Radiat Res 2012;177(4):449–66.

36. Abdulla S, Salavati A, Saboury B, et al. Quantitative assessment of global lung inflammation following radiation therapy using FDG PET/CT: a pilot study. Eur J Nucl Med Mol Imaging 2014;41(2):350–6.

37. Echeverria AE, McCurdy M, Castillo R, et al. Proton therapy radiation pneumonitis local dose-response in esophagus cancer patients. Radiother Oncol 2013;106(1):124–9.

38. Simone CB 2nd, Rengan R. The use of proton therapy in the treatment of lung cancers. Cancer J 2014;20(6):427–32.

39. Levin WP, Kooy H, Loeffler JS, et al. Proton beam therapy. Br J Cancer 2005;93(8):849–54.

40. Terasawa T, Dvorak T, Ip S, et al. Systematic review: charged-particle radiation therapy for cancer. Ann Intern Med 2009;151(8):556–65.

41. Kesarwala AH, Ko CJ, Ning H, et al. Intensity-modulated proton therapy for elective nodal irradiation and involved-field radiation in the definitive treatment of locally advanced non-small-cell lung cancer: a dosimetric study. Clin Lung Cancer 2015;16(3):237–44.

42. Wink KC, Roelofs E, Solberg T, et al. Particle therapy for non-small cell lung tumors: where do we stand? A systematic review of the literature. Front Oncol 2014;4:292.

43. Santoro F, Tarantino N, Pellegrino PL, et al. Cardiovascular sequelae of radiation therapy. Clin Res Cardiol 2014;103(12):955–67.

44. Adams MJ, Hardenbergh PH, Constine LS, et al. Radiation-associated cardiovascular disease. Crit Rev Oncol Hematol 2003;45(1):55–75.

45. Galper SL, Yu JB, Mauch PM, et al. Clinically significant cardiac disease in patients with Hodgkin lymphoma treated with mediastinal irradiation. Blood 2011;117(2):412–8.

46. Mauch PM, Kalish LA, Marcus KC, et al. Long-term survival in Hodgkin's disease relative impact of mortality, second tumors, infection, and cardiovascular disease. Cancer J Sci Am 1995;1(1):33–42.

47. Hancock SL, Tucker MA, Hoppe RT. Factors affecting late mortality from heart disease after treatment of Hodgkin's disease. JAMA 1993; 270(16):1949–55.

48. Aleman BM, van den Belt-Dusebout AW, De Bruin ML, et al. Late cardiotoxicity after treatment for Hodgkin lymphoma. Blood 2007; 109(5):1878–86.

49. Early Breast Cancer Trialists' Collaborative Group, Darby S, McGale P, et al. Effect of radiotherapy after breast-conserving surgery on 10-year recurrence and 15-year breast cancer death: meta-analysis of individual patient data for 10,801 women in 17 randomised trials. Lancet 2011; 378(9804):1707–16.

50. Cuzick J, Stewart H, Rutqvist L, et al. Cause-specific mortality in long-term survivors of breast cancer who participated in trials of radiotherapy. J Clin Oncol 1994;12(3):447–53.

51. Clarke M, Collins R, Darby S, et al. Effects of radiotherapy and of differences in the extent of surgery for early breast cancer on local recurrence and 15-year survival: an overview of the randomised trials. Lancet 2005;366(9503):2087–106.

52. Giordano SH, Kuo YF, Freeman JL, et al. Risk of cardiac death after adjuvant radiotherapy for breast cancer. J Natl Cancer Inst 2005;97(6):419–24.

53. Ragaz J, Olivotto IA, Spinelli JJ, et al. Locoregional radiation therapy in patients with high-risk breast cancer receiving adjuvant chemotherapy: 20-year results of the British Columbia randomized trial. J Natl Cancer Inst 2005;97(2):116–26.

54. Hojris I, Overgaard M, Christensen JJ, et al. Morbidity and mortality of ischaemic heart disease in high-risk breast-cancer patients after adjuvant postmastectomy systemic treatment with or without radiotherapy: analysis of DBCG 82b and 82c randomised trials. Radiotherapy Committee of the Danish Breast Cancer Cooperative Group. Lancet 1999;354(9188):1425–30.

55. Rutqvist LE, Lax I, Fornander T, et al. Cardiovascular mortality in a randomized trial of adjuvant radiation therapy versus surgery alone in primary breast cancer. Int J Radiat Oncol Biol Phys 1992;22(5): 887–96.

56. Rutter CE, Chagpar AB, Evans SB. Breast cancer laterality does not influence survival in a large modern cohort: implications for radiation-related cardiac mortality. Int J Radiat Oncol Biol Phys 2014; 90(2):329–34.

57. Killander F, Anderson H, Kjellén E, et al. Increased cardio and cerebrovascular mortality in breast cancer patients treated with postmastectomy radiotherapy–25 year follow-up of a randomised trial from the South Sweden Breast Cancer Group. Eur J Cancer 2014;50(13):2201–10.

58. Lally BE, Detterbeck FC, Geiger AM, et al. The risk of death from heart disease in patients with non-small cell lung cancer who receive postoperative radiotherapy: analysis of the surveillance, epidemiology, and end results database. Cancer 2007; 110(4):911–7.

59. Bradley JD, Paulus R, Komaki R, et al. Standard-dose versus high-dose conformal radiotherapy with concurrent and consolidation carboplatin plus paclitaxel with or without cetuximab for patients with stage IIIA or IIIB non-small-cell lung cancer (RTOG 0617): a randomised, two-by-two factorial phase 3 study. Lancet Oncol 2015;16(2):187–99.

60. Gholami S, Salavati A, Houshmand S, et al. Assessment of atherosclerosis in large vessel walls: a comprehensive review of FDG-PET/CT image acquisition protocols and methods for uptake quantification. J Nucl Cardiol 2015;22(3):468–79.

61. Fajardo LF, Stewart JR. Pathogenesis of radiation-induced myocardial fibrosis. Lab Invest 1973; 29(2):244–57.

62. Unal K, Unlu M, Akdemir O, et al. 18F-FDG PET/CT findings of radiotherapy-related myocardial changes in patients with thoracic malignancies. Nucl Med Commun 2013;34(9):855–9.

63. Zophel K, Hölzel C, Dawel M, et al. PET/CT demonstrates increased myocardial FDG uptake following irradiation therapy. Eur J Nucl Med Mol Imaging 2007;34(8):1322–3.

64. Jingu K, Kaneta T, Nemoto K, et al. The utility of 18F-fluorodeoxyglucose positron emission tomography for early diagnosis of radiation-induced myocardial damage. Int J Radiat Oncol Biol Phys 2006;66(3):845–51.

65. Evans JD, Gomez DR, Chang JY, et al. Cardiac (1)(8)F-fluorodeoxyglucose uptake on positron emission tomography after thoracic stereotactic body radiation therapy. Radiother Oncol 2013; 109(1):82–8.

66. Kallfass E, Kramling HJ, Schultz-Hector S. Early inflammatory reaction of the rabbit coeliac artery wall after combined intraoperative (IORT) and external (ERT) irradiation. Radiother Oncol 1996;39(2): 167–78.

67. Chen W, Bural GG, Torigian DA, et al. Emerging role of FDG-PET/CT in assessing atherosclerosis in large arteries. Eur J Nucl Med Mol Imaging 2009;36(1):144–51.

68. Wang YC, Hsieh TC, Chen SW, et al. Concurrent chemo-radiotherapy potentiates vascular inflammation: increased FDG uptake in head and neck cancer patients. JACC Cardiovasc Imaging 2013; 6(4):512–4.

69. Tofilon PJ, Fike JR. The radioresponse of the central nervous system: a dynamic process. Radiat Res 2000;153(4):357–70.

70. Schultheiss TE, Stephens LC. Invited review: permanent radiation myelopathy. Br J Radiol 1992; 65(777):737–53.

71. Sheline GE, Wara WM, Smith V. Therapeutic irradiation and brain injury. Int J Radiat Oncol Biol Phys 1980;6(9):1215–28.

72. Crossen JR, Garwood D, Glatstein E, et al. Neurobehavioral sequelae of cranial irradiation in adults: a review of radiation-induced encephalopathy. J Clin Oncol 1994;12(3):627–42.

73. Johannesen TB, Lien HH, Hole KH, et al. Radiological and clinical assessment of long-term brain tumour survivors after radiotherapy. Radiother Oncol 2003;69(2):169–76.

74. Giovagnoli AR, Boiardi A. Cognitive impairment and quality of life in long-term survivors of malignant brain tumors. Ital J Neurol Sci 1994;15(9):481–8.

75. Meyers CA, Brown PD. Role and relevance of neurocognitive assessment in clinical trials of patients with CNS tumors. J Clin Oncol 2006;24(8):1305–9.

76. Robbins ME, Bourland JD, Cline JM, et al. A model for assessing cognitive impairment after fractionated whole-brain irradiation in nonhuman primates. Radiat Res 2011;175(4):519–25.

77. Shaw EG, Rosdhal R, D'Agostino RB Jr, et al. Phase II study of donepezil in irradiated brain tumor patients: effect on cognitive function, mood, and quality of life. J Clin Oncol 2006;24(9):1415–20.

78. Baillieux H, De Smet HJ, Paquier PF, et al. Cerebellar neurocognition: insights into the bottom of the brain. Clin Neurol Neurosurg 2008;110(8):763–73.

79. Evans ES, Hahn CA, Kocak Z, et al. The role of functional imaging in the diagnosis and management of late normal tissue injury. Semin Radiat Oncol 2007;17(2):72–80.

80. Kahkonen M, Metsähonkala L, Minn H, et al. Cerebral glucose metabolism in survivors of childhood acute lymphoblastic leukemia. Cancer 2000;88(3):693–700.

81. Hahn CA, Zhou SM, Raynor R, et al. Dose-dependent effects of radiation therapy on cerebral blood flow, metabolism, and neurocognitive dysfunction. Int J Radiat Oncol Biol Phys 2009;73(4):1082–7.

82. Krull KR, Minoshima S, Edelmann M, et al. Regional brain glucose metabolism and neurocognitive function in adult survivors of childhood cancer treated with cranial radiation. J Nucl Med 2014;55(11):1805–10.

83. Chowhan NM. Injurious effects of radiation on the esophagus. Am J Gastroenterol 1990;85(2):115–20.

84. Kramer S, Gelber RD, Snow JB, et al. Combined radiation therapy and surgery in the management of advanced head and neck cancer: final report of study 73-03 of the Radiation Therapy Oncology Group. Head Neck Surg 1987;10(1):19–30.

85. Brucher BL, Weber W, Bauer M, et al. Neoadjuvant therapy of esophageal squamous cell carcinoma: response evaluation by positron emission tomography. Ann Surg 2001;233(3):300–9.

86. Flamen P, Van Cutsem E, Lerut A, et al. Positron emission tomography for assessment of the response to induction radiochemotherapy in locally advanced oesophageal cancer. Ann Oncol 2002;13(3):361–8.

87. Song SY, Kim JH, Ryu JS, et al. FDG-PET in the prediction of pathologic response after neoadjuvant chemoradiotherapy in locally advanced, resectable esophageal cancer. Int J Radiat Oncol Biol Phys 2005;63(4):1053–9.

88. Wieder HA, Brücher BL, Zimmermann F, et al. Time course of tumor metabolic activity during chemoradiotherapy of esophageal squamous cell carcinoma and response to treatment. J Clin Oncol 2004;22(5):900–8.

89. Brink I, Hentschel M, Bley TA, et al. Effects of neoadjuvant radio-chemotherapy on 18F-FDG-PET in esophageal carcinoma. Eur J Surg Oncol 2004;30(5):544–50.

90. Nijkamp J, Rossi M, Lebesque J, et al. Relating acute esophagitis to radiotherapy dose using FDG-PET in concurrent chemo-radiotherapy for locally advanced non-small cell lung cancer. Radiother Oncol 2013;106(1):118–23.

91. Yuan ST, Brown RK, Zhao L, et al. Timing and intensity of changes in FDG uptake with symptomatic esophagitis during radiotherapy or chemo-radiotherapy. Radiat Oncol 2014;9(1):37.

92. Oh D, Huh SJ. Insufficiency fracture after radiation therapy. Radiat Oncol J 2014;32(4):213–20.

93. Cooper KL, Beabout JW, Swee RG. Insufficiency fractures of the sacrum. Radiology 1985;156(1):15–20.

94. Peh WC, Gough AK, Sheeran T, et al. Pelvic insufficiency fractures in rheumatoid arthritis. Br J Rheumatol 1993;32(4):319–24.

95. Finiels H, Finiels PJ, Jacquot JM, et al. Fractures of the sacrum caused by bone insufficiency. Meta-analysis of 508 cases. Presse Med 1997;26(33):1568–73 [in French].

96. Tokumaru S, Toita T, Oguchi M, et al. Insufficiency fractures after pelvic radiation therapy for uterine cervical cancer: an analysis of subjects in a prospective multi-institutional trial, and cooperative study of the Japan Radiation Oncology Group (JAROG) and Japanese Radiation Oncology Study Group (JROSG). Int J Radiat Oncol Biol Phys 2012;84(2):e195–200.

97. Baxter NN, Habermann EB, Tepper JE, et al. Risk of pelvic fractures in older women following pelvic irradiation. JAMA 2005;294(20):2587–93.

98. Kwon JW, Huh SJ, Yoon YC, et al. Pelvic bone complications after radiation therapy of uterine cervical cancer: evaluation with MRI. AJR Am J Roentgenol 2008;191(4):987–94.

99. Uezono H, Tsujino K, Moriki K, et al. Pelvic insufficiency fracture after definitive radiotherapy for uterine cervical cancer: retrospective analysis of risk factors. J Radiat Res 2013;54(6):1102–9.

100. Oh D, Huh SJ, Nam H, et al. Pelvic insufficiency fracture after pelvic radiotherapy for cervical cancer: analysis of risk factors. Int J Radiat Oncol Biol Phys 2008;70(4):1183–8.

101. Ogino I, Okamoto N, Ono Y, et al. Pelvic insufficiency fractures in postmenopausal woman with advanced cervical cancer treated by radiotherapy. Radiother Oncol 2003;68(1):61–7.

102. Ikushima H, Osaki K, Furutani S, et al. Pelvic bone complications following radiation therapy of gynecologic malignancies: clinical evaluation of radiation-induced pelvic insufficiency fractures. Gynecol Oncol 2006;103(3):1100–4.

103. Park SH, Kim JC, Lee JE, et al. Pelvic insufficiency fracture after radiotherapy in patients with cervical cancer in the era of PET/CT. Radiat Oncol J 2011; 29(4):269–76.

104. Fayad LM, Cohade C, Wahl RL, et al. Sacral fractures: a potential pitfall of FDG positron emission tomography. AJR Am J Roentgenol 2003;181(5):1239–43.

105. Oh D, Huh SJ, Lee SJ, et al. Variation in FDG uptake on PET in patients with radiation-induced pelvic insufficiency fractures: a review of 10 cases. Ann Nucl Med 2009;23(6):511–6.

106. Ravenel JG, Gordon LL, Pope TL, et al. FDG-PET uptake in occult acute pelvic fracture. Skeletal Radiol 2004;33(2):99–101.

107. Tsuchida T, Kosaka N, Sugimoto K, et al. Sacral insufficiency fracture detected by FDG-PET/CT: report of 2 cases. Ann Nucl Med 2006;20(6):445–8.

108. Salavati A, Shah V, Wang ZJ, et al. F-18 FDG PET/CT findings in postradiation pelvic insufficiency fracture. Clin Imaging 2011;35(2):139–42.

109. Kato K, Aoki J, Endo K. Utility of FDG-PET in differential diagnosis of benign and malignant fractures in acute to subacute phase. Ann Nucl Med 2003; 17(1):41–6.

110. Simone CB 2nd, Ly D, Dan TD, et al. Comparison of intensity-modulated radiotherapy, adaptive radiotherapy, proton radiotherapy, and adaptive proton radiotherapy for treatment of locally advanced head and neck cancer. Radiother Oncol 2011; 101(3):376–82.

111. Cannon B, Schwartz DL, Dong L. Metabolic imaging biomarkers of postradiotherapy xerostomia. Int J Radiat Oncol Biol Phys 2012;83(5):1609–16.

112. Hakim SG, Jacobsen HCh, Hermes D, et al. Early immunohistochemical and functional markers indicating radiation damage of the parotid gland. Clin Oral Investig 2004;8(1):30–5.

113. Bussels B, Maes A, Flamen P, et al. Dose-response relationships within the parotid gland after radiotherapy for head and neck cancer. Radiother Oncol 2004;73(3):297–306.

114. Braam PM, Roesink JM, Moerland MA, et al. Long-term parotid gland function after radiotherapy. Int J Radiat Oncol Biol Phys 2005;62(3):659–64.

115. Eisbruch A, Kim HM, Terrell JE, et al. Xerostomia and its predictors following parotid-sparing irradiation of head-and-neck cancer. Int J Radiat Oncol Biol Phys 2001;50(3):695–704.

116. Roach MC, Turkington TG, Higgins KA, et al. FDG-PET assessment of the effect of head and neck radiotherapy on parotid gland glucose metabolism. Int J Radiat Oncol Biol Phys 2012;82(1):321–6.

117. Buus S, Grau C, Munk OL, et al. 11C-methionine PET, a novel method for measuring regional salivary gland function after radiotherapy of head and neck cancer. Radiother Oncol 2004;73(3): 289–96.

118. Rose BS, Liang Y, Lau SK, et al. Correlation between radiation dose to (1)(8)F-FDG-PET defined active bone marrow subregions and acute hematologic toxicity in cervical cancer patients treated with chemoradiotherapy. Int J Radiat Oncol Biol Phys 2012;83(4):1185–91.

119. Elicin O, Callaway S, Prior JO, et al. [(18)F]FDG-PET standard uptake value as a metabolic predictor of bone marrow response to radiation: impact on acute and late hematological toxicity in cervical cancer patients treated with chemoradiation therapy. Int J Radiat Oncol Biol Phys 2014;90(5): 1099–107.

120. McCurdy MR, Castillo R, Martinez J, et al. [18F]-FDG uptake dose-response correlates with radiation pneumonitis in lung cancer patients. Radiother Oncol 2012;104(1):52–7.

121. Petit SF, van Elmpt WJ, Oberije CJ, et al. [(1)(8)F] fluorodeoxyglucose uptake patterns in lung before radiotherapy identify areas more susceptible to radiation-induced lung toxicity in non-small-cell lung cancer patients. Int J Radiat Oncol Biol Phys 2011;81(3):698–705.

122. De Ruysscher D, Houben A, Aerts HJ, et al. Increased (18)F-deoxyglucose uptake in the lung during the first weeks of radiotherapy is correlated with subsequent radiation-induced lung toxicity (RILT): a prospective pilot study. Radiother Oncol 2009;91(3):415–20.

123. McCurdy M, Bergsma DP, Hyun E, et al. The role of lung lobes in radiation pneumonitis and radiation-induced inflammation in the lung: a retrospective study. J Radiat Oncol 2013;2(2):203–8.

124. Konski A, Li T, Christensen M, et al. Symptomatic cardiac toxicity is predicted by dosimetric and patient factors rather than changes in 18F-FDG PET determination of myocardial activity after chemoradiotherapy for esophageal cancer. Radiother Oncol 2012;104(1):72–7.

125. Dornfeld K, Hopkins S, Simmons J, et al. Posttreatment FDG-PET uptake in the supraglottic and glottic larynx correlates with decreased quality of life after chemoradiotherapy. Int J Radiat Oncol Biol Phys 2008;71(2):386–92.

Moving?

Make sure your subscription moves with you!

To notify us of your new address, find your **Clinics Account Number** (located on your mailing label above your name), and contact customer service at:

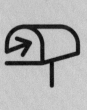

Email: journalscustomerservice-usa@elsevier.com

800-654-2452 (subscribers in the U.S. & Canada)
314-447-8871 (subscribers outside of the U.S. & Canada)

Fax number: 314-447-8029

Elsevier Health Sciences Division
Subscription Customer Service
3251 Riverport Lane
Maryland Heights, MO 63043

*To ensure uninterrupted delivery of your subscription, please notify us at least 4 weeks in advance of move.

Printed and bound by CPI Group (UK) Ltd, Croydon, CR0 4YY

03/10/2024

01040376-0009